Issues in Mental Health
Series Editor: Jo Campling

The care and status of persons with mental health problems has been identified as one of the key issues in health and society in the 1990s.

This series of books has been commissioned to give a multidisciplinary perspective: legal, medical, psychiatric and social work aspects of mental health will be covered. There is also an international perspective: wherever possible, books will compare developments in a range of different countries.

PUBLISHED

Philip Bean and Patricia Mounser
Discharged from Mental Hospitals

Suman Fernando
Mental Health, Race and Culture

Shulamit Ramon (editor)
Beyond Community Care: Normalisation and Integration Work

Shulamit Ramon
Mental Health in Europe

Anne Rogers, David Pilgrim and Ron Lacey
Experiencing Psychiatry: Users' Views of Services

FORTHCOMING

Philip Bean and Teresa Nemitz
Mental Health Law and Criminal Justice

The *Issues in Mental Health* series is published in association with:

MIND (National Association for Mental Health)
22 Harley Street, London W1N 2ED (0171–637–0741)

MIND is the leading mental health organisation in England and Wales. It works for a better life for people diagnosed, labelled or treated as mentally ill. It does this through campaigning, influencing government policy, training, education and service provision. Throughout its work MIND reflects its awareness of black and ethnic communities, and draws on the expertise of people with direct experience as providers and users of mental health services.

The points of view expressed in this publication do not necessarily reflect MIND policy.

Mental Health in Europe

Ends, Beginnings and Rediscoveries

Shulamit Ramon

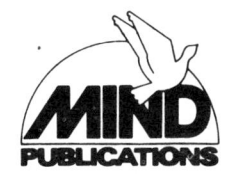

in association with

© Shulamit Ramon 1996

All rights reserved. No reproduction, copy or transmission of this publication may be made without written permission.

No paragraph of this publication may be reproduced, copied or transmitted save with written permission or in accordance with the provisions of the Copyright, Designs and Patents Act 1988, or under the terms of any licence permitting limited copying issued by the Copyright Licensing Agency, 90 Tottenham Court Road, London W1P 9HE.

Any person who does any unauthorised act in relation to this publication may be liable to criminal prosecution and civil claims for damages.

First published 1996 by
MACMILLAN PRESS LTD
Houndmills, Basingstoke, Hampshire RG21 6XS
and London
Companies and representatives
throughout the world

ISBN 0–333–59370–7 hardcover
ISBN 0–333–59371–5 paperback

A catalogue record for this book is available from the British Library.

10 9 8 7 6 5 4 3 2 1
05 04 03 02 01 00 99 98 97 96

Printed in Hong Kong

Published in the United States of America 1996 by
ST. MARTIN'S PRESS, INC.,
Scholarly and Reference Division
175 Fifth Avenue, New York, N.Y. 10010

ISBN 0–312–16066–6

Series Standing Order (Issues in Mental Health)

If you would like to receive future titles in this series as they are published, you can make use of our standing order facility. To place a standing order please contact your bookseller or, in case of difficulty, write to us at the address below with your name and address and the name of the series. Please state with which title you wish to begin your standing order. (If you live outside the United Kingdom we may not have the rights for your area, in which case we will forward your order to the publisher concerned.)

Customer Services Department, Macmillan Distribution Ltd
Houndmills, Basingstoke, Hampshire RG21 26S, England

This book is dedicated to the women and men still living in the psychiatric hospitals in Leros, and to those few Dutch, Greek and Italian professionals who are fighting against the odds of struggling psychiatric and social system.

It is also dedicated to **Amitai**: I hope that he grows up in a world in which Leros-type hospitals are a thing of the past.

Contents

List of Figures and Tables viii

Acknowledgements ix

Introduction 1

Prologue 8

1 Emerging Policy Perspectives 16

2 Conceptual Innovations 44

3 Ethnicity and Gender as Issues for Stakeholders in Mental Distress Services 73

4 Long-term Users of Mental Health Services 98

5 Innovations in Housing and Employment 136

6 Changing Professional Roles and Identities 160

7 A Scandalous Category: Media Representations of People Suffering from Mental Illness 186

Epilogue 211

References 213

Name Index 240

Subject Index 250

List of Figures and Tables

Figures

1.1 Rate of English hospital closure, 1960–2000   27
4.1 Involving service users in their own care management assessment   127

Tables

1   Recorded national rates of mental illness in 12 European countries   10
2   Suicide figures in 27 European countries and overall suicide rate, 1980–86   12
1.1 Number of beds in 10 European countries, 1980 and 1990   26
1.2 Community care costs by place of residence for people with mental health problems   38
2.1 Coping strategies when facing a threat to self-identity   47
3.1 Matrix of ethnicity and gender in the context of mental distress   74
4.1 Estimate of psychiatric outpatients with different diagnoses and number of visits in 1991   107

Acknowledgements

When preparing this book I was helped by too many people to name them all, as I progressively became very 'needy', especially in attempting to obtain updated information about non-hospital provisions and patterns of use of services in Europe. I got lost more than once in the process of writing this book by having to make sense of too much written information of one type and not enough of other types. Visiting real people, and services on the ground, was of immense help in enabling me to refocus.

I would therefore like to thank warmly my hosts in Greece (especially in Leros), Hungary, Italy (especially in Pordenone, Prato, Trieste and Turin), Kiev, Lujblijana, the Netherlands, Moscow and Portugal.

SHULAMIT RAMON

Introduction

I began to write this introduction at the end of 1993 when I had just come back from a journey that took me to Turin (in Italy) and Kiev (in Ukraine). In Turin we were celebrating the achievements of Italian psychiatric reformers in Grulisaco and Colegno, two large ex-hospitals on the outskirts of that metropolis, with a conference entitled Recomincare di Essere (Re-beginning to Be). In Kiev we were visiting psychiatric facilities as part of a fact-finding tour aimed at establishing social work in Ukraine, as one step towards reforming Ukrainian psychiatry and society.

It is all too easy to point out the numerous differences between Italy and Ukraine, and their mental health systems. On the surface there is little similarity between the two systems. Yet what seems to unite the activists in the two systems is the *quest for a fresh start*, in which the lessons of the past are learned for the purpose of establishing better systems. The primary objective of this book is to contribute to this process in each of the European mental health systems, as we approach the end of the twentieth century and prepare ourselves for the twenty-first century. This objective entails:

1. Providing an overview of the major developments and processes that have taken place in European mental health systems since 1980.
2. Contextualising these developments within the social, political, cultural and economic layers of our existence in which these events and processes have occurred.
3. Analysing the significance of these developments for those involved in mental health systems.
4. Indicating potential future paths.

Why focus on Europe?

The majority of publications with a comparative perspective on mental health either originate in the United States, or look to it as their ideal. Indeed the United States has been the initiator of far-reaching changes in the approach to mental health in the post Second World War period. Some of the best – and some of the worst – ideas, policies, services and organisations exist there. A lot has been written about its mental health system systems, and a lot remains to be learned and discussed.

Europe is moving towards becoming a single political entity within the European Union (EU), with an expanding membership, and it is becoming urgent for Europeans throughout the EU and outside to know what is taking place in different member countries so that they may learn from each other and collaborate in the development of an improved system.

Furthermore the dominance of the North American influence has perhaps stifled the debate and narrowed its scope, where a far-ranging debate and a widening of options are much needed. While we have been overexposed to the North American influence, we have been considerably underexposed to information on the various European systems, which will form the basis of joint and separate decisions within the EU and by individual member states, as well as with and by non-member countries. Very few existing texts provide such a perspective,[1] and none of them include developments that have taken place between 1990 and 1995. These texts – and the many articles published in between – have been useful and have whetted our appetite to learn more about the situation Europe. However they have included little that relates to non-traditional stakeholders' perspective, and have provided insufficient in-depth analysis of the content and processes of change.

It is impossible to provide a comprehensive coverage of all developments in European mental health systems from 1980 onward in one volume. The scale of the variations in mental distress itself precludes such a task from being successfully completed. Instead this book is structured to cover a number of central themes, within which a *comparative perspective* is given, usually pertaining to not more than three countries per theme. Thus the text is selective from the outset. Deciding which themes to include and which to exclude was a difficult task. The final selection was directed primarily by consideration of which areas have seen more far-reaching developments since 1980, without attempting to judge which mental health aspect is more important, and not assuming that there have been no developments in aspects not covered in this book. Inevitably such a judgement is coloured by the author's knowledge and values, leaving space for others to add their contributions.

This book focuses on:

- Long-term adult users of mental health services and their relatives (excluding dementia suffers). Although relatively few in comparison with all users of mental health systems (though not few in number), they constitute the *major rediscovery* of the 1980–95 period.
- The interaction between policies, key social and psychological factors, beliefs, concepts, structures and methods of working with these people.
- The emergence of new stakeholders.
- The impact of new developments on established and emerging stakeholders.

The information presented in this book has been taken from official and research publications on each theme, media coverage, impressions formed during visits and revisits to a number of European mental health systems, talking to stakeholders and reading what they have written, and from knowledge gained in my capacity as researcher, educator, participant in policy-changing networks and member of both professional and user-focused organisations. Thus personal experience figures in this book as much as analysis and observation.

To prepare for this book I have recently visited Greece, Hungary, Italy, the Netherlands, Portugal, Russia, Slovenia and Ukraine. Previously I visited mental health facilities in Belgium, Czechoslovakia, Denmark, France, Germany, Finland and Spain. An in-depth knowledge of the systems in Britain (where I live and work) and Italy (whose psychiatric reform I have been investigating since 1981), coupled with several visits to mental health facilities in the United States and an up-to-date knowledge of the American literature, as well as recent visits to Japanese and Brazilian mental health facilities, have helped me to render intelligible other European systems.

Concerning change, the two main questions to be investigated in this book are:

- Has the considerable change in the 1980s and 1990s led to *fundamental* changes in the aims and modes of operation of these systems, or not?

- Have the changes been positive for the major stakeholders, or not?

Deciding whether changes are positive or negative depend on ethical beliefs pertaining to mental illness, the people who suffer from it, their relatives and friends, judgement as to degrees of risk, vulnerability and harm, as well as the place of mental health services in the pecking order of priorities within the context of welfare services. High on my own list of positive achievements are developments that are guided by the following ethics:

- People suffering from mental distress should be respected as individuals.
- They should be given the right to make decisions concerning their lives, and be provided with full information on the different options available to them. Only in extreme conditions should decisions be taken by others on their behalf.
- They should be offered a safe, supportive and respectful non-hospital environment in the event of a mental distress crisis.
- Housing, income assurance, participation in social networks and employment constitute basic needs and desires, and therefore should be an undeniable part of individual rights in European societies.
- Others involved should likewise be offered support and a guarantee of safety.
- There is no place for discrimination within mental health systems on the basis of age, class, colour, ethnicity, gender, nationality or religion.
- Professional intervention should be as minimal as possible, but when required should be the best available.
- All services should have in-built quality assurance measures that are made explicit and have been constructed with the involvement of users and carers.
- Solidarity, mutual support and advocacy should form an integral part of the rationale of mental health services.

While not excluding the potential usefulness of a clinical–somatic approach when relevant, this text is more influenced by psychosocial approaches and its author takes a critical stance towards the dominance of the first of these approaches in European mental health systems. It is encouraging to note that some psychiatrists are also coming to this conclusion. Thus McCrone and Strathdee suggested recently:

> There are clear indications that among clinicians, patterns of diagnostic assessment are changing. For example, as Leff (1992) indicates, the use of the term schizophrenia is essentially in itself inaccurate and covers a range of heterogenous conditions, which are themselves difficult to define clearly.... There are clear indications that diagnosis does not predict patterns of symptom complexes, prognosis or treatment effectiveness and therefore resource needs. The futility of diagnosis as the main variable in this context has been detailed above. Two recent fields of interest suggest the direction for future development, the determination of individual needs in case management service programmes and service use as a proxy for need.[2]

If diagnosis is an obstacle to providing good services – as argued since the 1960s by sociologists, social workers, psychologists and some psychiatrists, but dismissed by the psychiatric establishment – then the dominance of medication as the most prevalent method of intervention needs urgently to be questioned too.

Claude Louzoun,[3] heading the European research group on human rights in mental health systems, has recently suggested that a 'white' book of psychiatry be prepared. Such a book would commemorate the following:

- In the 1980s and the 1990s we have witnessed in Europe the closure of a number of psychiatric hospitals, and a considerable reduction in periods of hospitalisation.
- The resettlement in the community of the long-stay residents of these hospitals.
- The creation of users' and carers' organisations.
- The establishment of a variety of services in the community, including some that are run by carers and users, by women for women and by ethnic minority members for ethnic minorities.
- The legislation of more liberal mental health laws that provide more assurances of human rights.
- Instances of reintegration of people with serious mental illness into mainstream ordinary living settings.
- The rediscovery of continued care clients as people rather then patients.

- The usefulness of medication has been questioned and alternatives sought.
- Greater flexibility on the part of some professionals.
- Greater readiness on the part of the general public and politicians to have people with serious mental illness in our midst.

The other side of the balance sheet will show:

- The opening of new, private, for-profit psychiatric hospitals and clinics.
- Homeless people becoming sufferers of mental illness, and the homelessness of people with serious mental illness.
- The continued spending of most mental health budgets on hospitals rather than on non-hospital services.
- The near total absence of asylum facilities in the community.
- Pressure to legislate for compulsory treatment in the community.
- Demonisation of the continued care client (especially those who refuse to take medication).
- Continued overuse of the more coercive and chemical means of intervention with members of black ethnic minorities, working-class people, and women.
- The rigidity of many professionals.
- The continuing fear of some members of the general public and politicians to have people with serious mental illnesses in their midst.

The list could be made longer, but I hope that the point of acknowledging the changes as well as their contradictory nature has been convincingly made.

As part of the new trend, a number of European networks have emerged in the field of mental health, including a users' network, the European Mental Health Regional network as part of the Council of Europe, and a European network of professionals and researchers within the World Health Organisation (WHO). These networks are only one reflection of the much greater impact the EU has had on all Western European mental health systems, as well as on most other social systems, since 1980. Its impact on ex-communist countries is more indirect, but has increased since 1989, as will be described in Chapter 2.

The effect of living in 'the global village' extends beyond the impact of the EU to that of the global economic climate, especially the impact of US mental health policies in the post-welfare-state era. These too will be looked at in Chapter 2.

While in a post-modern world it is fashionable to focus on differences rather than similarities among and within societies, it will be suggested here that perhaps the degree of similarity is greater than is usually acknowledged. Likewise the *applicability* of ideas and principles of action originating in one European country to the rest of Europe is greater than is usually accepted. A flippant 'it won't work here', uttered without examination when confronted with an innovation coming from another country, is usually a defensive reaction, made by those who are happy with the *status quo*.

Of course each innovation requires careful consideration prior to adoption within and between countries, yet all too often both blissful and wilful ignorance exist side by side with misinterpretation of anything perceived as 'foreign'. While mental distress and psychiatry are assumed to have universal validity, the behaviour of the mental health team in the next neighbourhood is perceived as 'odd' if different from that of our own team, let alone that of another country in which people speak another language. The behaviour of the other team may indeed be odd; it may also be more beneficial to clients then ours, or less so. In any case it should be known to us, looked into and its usefulness to our situation evaluated.

Inevitably, such a high degree of change also entails a high degree of uncertainty, confusion and anxiety. This book attempts to clear away some of the mist by enabling the reader to be better informed and by indicating the *central and essential* elements of the changing systems. Faced with so many ends, new beginnings and rediscoveries, this is a most exciting exhausting, challenging and baffling period for anyone interested in European mental health systems.

I hope that the book will be part of the reader's journey into the unfolding story of the recent past, the current present, the near and far future of these systems and their stakeholders.

SHULAMIT RAMON

Prologue: Mental Health, Distress and Illness-Social Constructs, 'Facts' and Figures

As our journey into European mental health systems begins, it is necessary to be as clear as possible about what is meant by mental health, distress and illness. It would also be useful to know beforehand about the scope of the phenomena discussed in this text.

At the risk of repeating a truism, I shall state from the outset that there is no agreement as to what constitutes mental health, distress or illness, neither between the main stakeholders in this field, nor within the scientific disciplines preoccupied with it. Mainstream psychiatry defines mental health as the absence of illness, and the latter as a disruption in ordinary functioning expressed by a set of symptoms that typify a specific diagnostic category that is likely to be caused by underlying biological factors, triggered off at times by psychological and social factors.[1] As early as 1958, Marie Jahoda[2] proposed six components of mental health, focused on maintaining the duality of personal autonomy and adjustment to social life. In Asian religions mental health is defined as achieving harmony within the world, especially with nature, whereas psychoanalysis defined as achieving a balance between love and work, or between pleasure and a disciplined interaction with others.[3]

There is a greater degree of agreement on the definition of mental illness as a disruption in ordinary functioning than on any of the other components mentioned above. The significance of symptoms, and the unusual behaviour, feelings and thoughts that at times accompany the appearance of symptoms, as well as the in underlying causes, are all hotly disputed by different stakeholders and disciplines. The suffering experienced by the individual, and by those close to her/him, is the only other element that is not disputed, though its significance is. As we also lack agreement as to the validity of the evidence accumulated by the different protagonists, it can be concluded that mental health, distress and illness are *social constructs* that depend on the particular interpretation of the main actors in a specific situation.

A vast literature and body of research exists on the issue of how we – lay people and professionals – form social constructs.[4] It highlights the fact that at times we form social representations that contain ambiguity and contradictory elements, and not only consistent and congruous ideas. This in turn implies that facts and figures in this field need to be treated carefully, with a good understanding of the definitions underlying their collection, as with different definitions not only are different facts collected, but the same figures acquire a different meaning.

There is no available statistical coverage on mental health in Europe. At best, statistical knowledge of mental distress and illness in Europe can be described as inadequate. This is due not only to the lack of agreement as to what mental distress and illness mean. It also derives from the lack of a European umbrella organisation to collate the figures regularly and the different methods of collecting them in different countries, as well data not being collected in the first place (because of inefficiency, not seeing it as important, or due to political considerations).

Most of the available figures have been collected according to definitions provided by mainstream psychiatry; hence the strengths and weaknesses of the data relate to the dominance of the clinical–somatic model of mental distress. Doubts about the validity and reliability of psychiatric diagnosis in principle have been expressed, some of which are echoed in Chapter 2. Concern about validity and reliability concerning specific groups in the population, such as members of ethnic minorities and women, are reflected in Chapter 3.

Wherever relevant and available, statistical information will be presented throughout the text. Table 1 represents the latest attempt (1993) by the Council of Europe to put together figures on mental illness in Europe.

Table 1 highlights the many gaps in the statistical information available in Western Europe on the rates of mental illness. However the table masks the fact that the statistics presented are likely to have been collected in more than one way, and therefore doubts about their validity are justified. It would be interesting to know why such statistics have not been collated, or whether they are recorded as part of general medical statistics. As it is, the lack of data does not facilitate good planning.

Table 1 Recorded national rates of mental illness in 12 European countries (per 1000 people)

Country	General (Populat. care)	Primary	Specialised (Out-patient)	Hospital
Belgium	—	—	—	—
Denmark (Malmo)	19.4	—	—	43.9
Finland	120.0	—	30.0	6.9
Ireland	—	—	24.3	85.4
Italy	—	—	—	—
Norway	200.0	200	67.0	9.0
Portugal	17.0	—	—	—
Spain	—	—	—	—
Sweden	40.0	340	25.0	—
UK	—	140	6.0	1.7

Note: Dashes denote a lack of nationally recorded figures.
Source: Council of Europe, *European cooperation concerning epidemiological studies in the field of mental health* (Strasbourg: Council of Europe, 1993, pp. 22–34.

The British Mental Health Foundation has estimated that in the UK 6 000 000 people suffer from mental distress, that is, about 10 per cent of the general population, of whom about 60 000 are inpatients.[5] Based on this figure, a rough estimate of the twelve member states of the EU, where there are about 300 million inhabitants, implies that about 30 million have suffered from mental distress, most of them of mild forms, while about three million have suffered from serious mental distress.

To illustrate the complexity of combining social constructs with facts and figures, a brief analysis of the findings based on a WHO European research project on suicide and attempted suicide will be presented here. The project took place throughout the 1980s and was aimed at gaining an accurate picture of the phenomenon of suicide and attempted suicide (in terms of prevalence, mode, related social and personal factors) in order to design an improved intervention scheme. Researchers from most Western European countries participated, with the occasional East European contribution. Numerous publications came out of it, the most comprehensive being the edited texts by Platt and Krietman,[6] Diekstra *et al.*[7] and Crepet *et al.*[8]

Suicide, which led to the death of 135 000 people in Europe in 1989,[9] and attempted suicide (430 000 attempts in the same year) deserve our attention on a number of grounds. Suicide on this scale:

- reflects the high level of misery experienced by a large number of individuals, their relatives and friends;
- implies that a large number of people are unable to function normally;
- uses vast resources in terms of medical and social personnel, hospital beds, medication, counselling and psychotherapy;
- the relatively high level of repeated episodes of attempted suicide implies that there is place for improving our methods of intervention.

Before turning to the information collated as part of the project (Table 2), it is important to remember that suicide may be attempted as part of a state of mental illness, but also without any such state being identified. Yet we would be justified in arguing that any person attempting suicide is suffering from mental distress, that is, from emotional and psychological suffering. Hence the decision to approach suicide as a mental health issue comes out of constructing it socially as such.

When collecting evidence on these issues we are aware that different cultural traditions and their approach to suicide will to an extent determine whether or not a death, or a self-harm attempt, is described as suicide. Thus a further element of social construction creeps into the first phases of creating an epidemiological base.

Table 2 highlights that on the whole the rates correspond to the figures, but not fully, mainly because male and female suicide figures do not follow the same pattern from one country to the other. For example Finland has the second highest number in terms of male suicide, but only the sixth in terms of female suicide. The (then) Federal Republic of Germany had the second highest overall rate of suicide, but was the second lowest in terms of female suicide and eighth in terms of male suicide.

Furthermore the rate changed in most countries between 1960 and 1986, usually towards a significantly increased rate. The case of Hungary, which topped the list for all indicators in 1986 and had the second highest rate in 1960, will be used for the purpose of further explanation. According to Harmat[10] Hungary has had the highest suicide vale in the world since 1968. Under

Table 2 Suicide figures in 27 European countries and overall suicide rate, 1980–86 (per 100 000)

Country	Males	Females	Overall (1960)	Rate (1980–6)
Hungary	661	259	25.0	45.3
Germany (F.R)	266	92	37.0	43.1
Germany (D.R)	n.a	n.a	28.6	19.0
Austria	421	158	23.1	28.3
Denmark	351	206	20.3	27.8
Finland	430	113	20.5	26.6
Belgium	330	153	14.6	23.8
Switzerland	326	132	29.2	22.8
France	331	127	15.8	22.7
Czechoslovakia	292	92	22.3	18.9
Sweden	250	115	17.4	18.5
Bulgaria	232	94	8.7	16.3
Yugoslavia	228	97	13.9	16.1
Norway	208	74	6.4	14.1
Luxembourg	207	74	13.4	13.9
Iceland	206	58	10.6	13.3
Poland	220	44	8.0	13.0
Scotland	166	60	7.9	11.6
Netherlands	146	81	6.6	11.0
N.Ireland	131	39	4.4	9.3
Portugal	136	51	8.7	9.2
England & Wales	121	57	10.6	8.9
Ireland	92	39	4.4	7.8
Italy	110	43	6.1	7.6
Spain	68	23	5.5	4.9
Greece	57	25	4.3	4.1
Malta	n.a	6	0.9	0.1

Note: n.a = not available.
Sources: figures: WHO Statistics Annual, 1987; rates: WHO Data Bank, July 1988.

the harshest phase of political and economic oppression the rate dropped considerably (to 21.5 in 1950–54), and has been levelling off, but still at a high level, since 1983. Suicide is particularly high among older people (65 plus) and younger people in the 15–24 age group. There are no significant differences in the suicide rate between urban and rural areas, or between members of the Catholic and Protestant Churches since 1945. Those who are widowed or divorced, and without children have a higher rate of suicide. Although more men commit suicide than women, Hungarian women have the highest rate of suicide among European women.

Hungary has been much less deprived economically and less oppressed politically than a number of other European countries. It does not have a particularly high rate of *identified* mental illness. The explanation provided by Hungarians themselves for the high incidence of suicide is twofold:

1. A number of creative, well-respected people, have committed suicide, and therefore *culturally* suicide is perceived as a socially acceptable solution for people who feel that they have excluded the end of that entrance, both psychologically and socially.
2. Supportive social networks have diminished in number and effectiveness due to political and social instability, an explanation that follows the classical conceptual framework developed much earlier by Durkheim,[11] centred on the concept of anomie.

Further predictors of an increase in national rates of suicide include an increase in the divorce rate, a decrease in the number of young people, high unemployment and a high rate of homicide.[12] These too are expressions of anomie.

While attempted suicide is perceived as the best predictor of completed suicide,[13] followed by alcohol misuse, the *gender* correlation is inverted in suicide attempts. A ratio of two attempts by women to one attempt by men, or higher, is reported.[14] Nevertheless, with the exception of the study by Jack,[15] rarely does the research focus on gender in either suicide or attempted suicide, apart from looking at the *methods* of self-harm (that is, more men use violent methods, more women use less violent methods).

A higher proportion of people with an identified mental illness also take to self-harm, particularly those suffering from depression and schizophrenia, where the reported rates of suicide are either twice or thrice the rate of the general population.[16] It has been claimed that people diagnosed as having an 'inadequate personality' also have a high rate of suicide and suicide attempts.[17] More recently, however, it has been suggested that such people may be simply depressed.[18] However all of this pales into insignificance when compared with the rate of suicide among people with alcohol addiction, which is about nine times higher than that of the general population.[19]

On the face of it, what unites people with diagnosed depression, schizophrenia, inadequate personality and alcohol addiction is *despair*, a *sense of failure* and *loss of direction*. These feelings are also coming across in descriptions of people who have self-harmed without being diagnosed as suffering from an identified mental illness.[20] It would therefore seem that we are faced with two dichotomous possibilities:

1. To perceive and treat everyone who has attempted suicide as mentally ill, because such a transgression of acceptable social ethics and norms cannot otherwise be understood.
2. To perceive and treat such people as experiencing a generalised sense of despair and lack of control and purpose, triggered by an adverse life event, in which a suicide attempt is a cry for help and a completed suicide is an at of escape and revenge.

While most psychiatrists have opted for the first of these, sociologists, social workers and psychologists have often opted for the second. The latter have looked not only at the concept of anomie mentioned above, but also at hopelessness[21] and attribution theory.[22] The explanatory framework is of considerable importance not only in making sense of a behaviour experienced by all of us as uncomfortable, shocking or scandalous, but also in enabling us to identify the type of intervention that is most likely to be of use for people at risk of attempting suicide, or after an unsuccessful attempt.

The vast literature on intervention and prevention will not be summarised here; although some of it will be looked at in Chapter 5, which focuses on the continued care clients of mental health services (the reader specifically interested in intervention methods can look these up in the three texts that summarise the European WHO project, mentioned above). The impact on relatives and friends will be looked at in part in Chapters 3 and 5, whereas the impact on workers will be discussed in Chapter 7.

Thus suicide and attempted suicide cross-cut a number of central issues for mental health systems and services, as well as demonstrate the benefits and limitations of the use of facts and figures. Above all the study of these phenomena highlights the interwoven relationships between social construction and the methods of operationalising such constructions into units that lead to the collection of specific – and highly selective – information, which is in turn used for the reconstruction of our understanding and reaction to suicide.

1
Emerging Policy Perspectives

Mental health policies form an integral part of social policies concerning marginalised groups in society. Marginalisation refers in this case to a high degree of stigmatisation and relative poverty, being in need of social support above the ordinary during periods of inability to function at the same level as others, resulting in social powerlessness.[1] This is also reflected in the marginality of mental health policies within the study of social policy as a discipline. Most general texts on social policy do not even mention this area, and usually just have a short section entitled 'the disabled' or 'elderly and disabled people'.[2]

Policies are important not only as a reflection of dominant public opinion, but also as pointers to preferred service structures and interventions. As with any other policy, such policies are influenced by political, cultural and economic ideologies and facts created by the interplay of these factors. To make sense of the development and impact of mental health policies, we need to understand:

- the processes by which social policies are made;
- the political, cultural and economic contexts in which policy decisions are taken.

Legislation is perceived here as reflecting policy preferences. Therefore relevant laws will be looked at within the context of a specific policy, rather than being separated out.

Processes of state policy formation

Often, decisions are described by policy analysts as the result of logical and intellectual reasoning; others focus on political motivation and objectives as the main underlying logic.[3]

There is little evidence to suggest that governments seriously consider policy options that do not serve them politically, or that a debate on options is initiated without entertaining a number of prejudices, some of which are political. More then one motive may play a part, hence policy decisions are likely to reflect ambiguities and at times contradictions, rather then the clear-cut sloganised version that is put forward for propaganda purposes. Therefore governments are influenced by more groups and factors than they would perhaps like to admit. Within a parliamentary democracy, debates in parliament are one arena for the expression of different opinions and policy options.

In addition to other ideological influences, recently European governments have often demonstrated that they are primarily influenced by *economic* considerations, specifically cost-cutting rather than cost-effectiveness. While this motive can be detected in some policies, the opposite seems to be true of others (for example, despite the stated preference for providing community mental health facilities, financial resources continue to be invested predominately in beds in all European countries), thus puncturing the myths that governments would have us believe in. Instead, most governments find it difficult to get rid of the impact of past policies and they bow to vested interest groups perceived as powerful, such as the medical profession, insurance companies and elements of the media.

A related utilitarian motive attributed to government policy thinking is that of *efficiency*, namely the rational and effective use of available resources. While the desire of governments to close hospitals that are already half empty can be understood as a drive for efficiency, the apparent blindness to the processes required for a successful psychiatric hospital closure in terms of staff sensitivity and use of existing staff belie this myth too as an oversimplistic explanation.[4]

The media is playing an increasing and crucial role in focusing on some options while discarding others, but without logical consideration or debate. As Chapter 7 will demonstrate, the media not only pushes for some options, but also reflects meanings provided from elsewhere, thus rendering intelligible material that would otherwise be bothersome for its lack of immediate coherence. The underlying reasons for choice of option in the media are influenced by the ideological and political positions of editors and journalists, but also by assumptions about what will captivate their audience.

Governments are also influenced by professionals working in a particular field, though in mental health there is a recognisable hierarchy of professional influence that corresponds to the social status of the medical profession in our society. Within the general lay population some groups are more influential than others, either because they are the mainstay of the party in power or because they have managed to influence the media, becoming noticed by the government in this way. As we will see in Chapters 4 and 7, relatives of people suffering from serious mental illness are one such group in a number of European countries.

Given the number of influencing factors and groups, it is understandable that changes in policy are often demanded from governments rather than being initiated by them. The reactive nature of most governments implies that long-term policies are rarely waiting in the wings to be picked up at the right political moment in the field of mental health. A government will listen selectively to the views of different pressure groups and will tend to choose the option that requires the least change from existing policies and structures.[5]

At times this may not be possible, as pressure from specific quarters may be perceived as too dominant or may have much greater political appeal than other choices. These are the instances in which *radical change* may be embarked upon, which may or may not be more expensive than less glamorous options.[6] A favoured alternative is the choice that appears to be radical, but is not so in reality. The registering of people deemed to be suffering from serious mental illness and to be at risk, legislated by the British government in April 1994, provides a cogent example of this tactic – apparently some hospitals are refusing to implement it as the cost of doing so is high (the *Independent*, 14 July 1994) and the benefits are no different from those already possible without the register. Yet due to pressure from the media and relatives' organisations the British government felt it had to do something that would look like a radical move to remedy a chaotic situation.

The above example reflects another instance that may facilitate more fundamental change, namely if the government sees itself to be in a *legitimation crisis*[7] in which its authority to make decisions is questioned either in general or in relation to a specific area. Given the sensitivity of the public and the media to mental illness issues, a series of scandals can rock the boat of legitimacy of the government and/or experts in this field. Mechanisms of response to a legitimation crisis are illustrated by the reaction of the post-1989 Romanian government to the exposure of inhuman conditions in children's homes and hospitals. It allowed the WHO and Unicef to establish a mental health task force whose main roles were to gather information on mental health services, make policy recommendations and act upon the latter.[8]

Similarly, but on a different scale and without outside intervention, the British government set up a mental health task force, to operate for for two years (December 1992–1994), to ensure that the radical changes it wished to impose on mental health services would be promoted and sustained. The task force had a small number of paid staff, headed by one non-civil-servant ex-health-service manager who had directed one of the more successful hospital closures in Britain. Unlike the US mental health task force, which had an advisory role, the British task force had the authority to initiate and operationalise changes.

Within the task force was a core group who represented different stakeholders (users, health service directors, social services directors and carers) and a larger support group with representatives from the voluntary sector, the mental health professions and related organisations. Apart from periodic meetings in which issues of a general nature were aired with the aim of providing blueprint guidance, the task force also:

- Generated ten user conferences across the country.

- Initiated a monthly newsletter entitled *Water Towers*, the title of the famous speech made by Enoch Powell, minister of health in 1962, calling for the closure of Victorian psychiatric hospitals; and a publication entitled *Grassroots*, which focuses on examples of innovative good practice.

- Provided about 100 one-off grants ranging from £5000 to £25 000 for innovative projects in existing services. Each member of the task force support group was asked to support one such project, together with one of the paid staff members. The nature and extent of the support was left to the supporter.

- Contracted two teams of consultants on a short-term basis to provide evidence on the scope of closure and reprovision, and the quality of these services.

- Contracted a consultant for six months to recommend and initiate innovative services for black ethnic minorities.

- Contracted an outside consultant to devise a framework for a

comprehensive service, mainly through library research and reliance on the US experience and service examples. European experiences and service models were ruled out as irrelevant.
- Provided an emergency assessment of the state of the services offered in London, culminating in a very conservative list of recommendations that contradicted the general stance taken by the task force (for example calling for more beds rather than for crisis and asylum facilities).

It is too early to evaluate the usefulness of this interesting and innovative experiment. Its curious mixture of encouraging innovation from above by supporting disempowered groups such as service users, small-scale support for purchasers and providers already committed to the changes, while putting less emphasis on influencing the bulk of service purchasers or providers was unusual. Whether this was sufficient to meet the scheme's objectives remains to be seen.

The context

Considerable changes have taken place in Europe since 1980, which will be summarised here. Politically we have witnessed the end of communism and the emergence of nationalism, of large states splitting into smaller units (for example Yugoslavia). The eruption of war between some of these newly created states, and the resulting huge number of refugees, injuries and fatalities has considerable implications for mental health provision.

The expansion of the EU into a political entity is important in terms of mental health, despite the lack of specifically targeted policies or action programmes that focus on mental distress. The EU has a stated commitment to protect vulnerable groups in each of the member states, mainly through the activities of individual members. General programmes that have focused on improving access to and the quality of education, women's welfare, social security and pensions have also benefited individuals suffering from mental distress.[9]

Some of programmes taking place within the broad remit of the Social Chapter – such as the social exclusion and poverty programme, the vocational rehabilitation programme and the disability programme – have also benefited people suffering from mental illness, albeit in a limited way. Some member states have taken advantage of these programmes to expand and change their mental health services. For example Italy has made extensive used of the vocational rehabilitation schemes to introduce work and training schemes for people suffering from mental distress, unlike Britain.[10]

In one unique case, that of Greece, the EU has committed eight million ECU since 1984 towards the restructuring of its mental health services (EC, Regulation 815, 1984). This followed the exposure of the inhuman and degrading conditions in the psychiatric hospitals on Leros, and the dire state of the services nationally (for a fuller description of the programme see Madianos and Yfantopolous.[11] The programme included the introduction of community mental health centres, the provision of extra psychiatric wards in general hospitals, and improving the conditions of existing mental hospitals and resettling their inpatients. Of these four components only the second seems to have been pursued seriously and successfully by the Greek government. While 33 new psychiatric wards have been established in general hospitals, only 10 community mental health centres have been created, despite the fact that they are a lot less expensive to establish in the first place. The very mixed aftermath of the programme in Leros is described in Chapter 5.

For quality assurance purposes the EU has sent a team of inspectors every three months. The inspectors come from a number of other EU countries and are mostly psychiatrists or well-known figures in the voluntary sector. Although the inspectors have been under considerable pressure not to rock the boat, the programme has been twice stopped and restarted, due to to-ing and fro-ing between the Greek government and the inspectors. The inspectors have no power over the Greek government, and it would seem that the EU too has no such power, apart from being able to suspend the programme. This state of affairs highlights the delicate balance between a member state and the central authority of EU institutions in the field of mental health.

Two umbrella organisations have been established relatively recently under the auspices of the EU: the European region of the Wared Mental Health Federation (WMHF) as part of the Council of Europe, and the European users network. Operating with no more than symbolic budgets, the two organisations are attempting to create European alliances to promote what they see as positive initiatives in different member states. So far their activities have been restricted to conferences and publications. Neither organisation has a clear policy position and they are yet to prove their worth. Their very existence, however, can be seen as a sign that the EU recognises mental illness as a social problem and is taking the position that service users, the most marginalised group, deserve its support.

Economically we seem to have been living through a permanent crisis since 1973, regardless of a few years of economic prosperity in the early 1980s. The crisis has resulted in growing unemployment, poverty and homelessness across Europe.[12] Many European governments have moved ideologically towards the idea of a market economy,[13] and have shifted their welfare policies accordingly. This shift in welfare policies has meant a move from a universal to a more residual provision of services more stringent eligibility criteria and persistent cuts in public sector spending. A more mixed welfare economy is favoured, where the not-for-profit and for-profit service sectors are encouraged to expand at the expense of the public service sector.

An example of the radical restructuring of welfare services having a direct impact on the users of mental health services is provided by the British 1990 NHS (national health service) and Community Care Act. The application of the law involved the following:

- The purchase and provision of units, each of which is run as a *business unit*, that is, it has to balance its books at the end of each budgetary year and is not allowed to carry a deficit from one year to the next.
- The introduction of *trust units*, that is, services are run as autonomous units within the larger service and take with them capital that previously belonged to that larger unit (for example a health district).
- General Practitioners (family doctors) are being encouraged by the government to become budget holders for all the services provided to their patients.
- The non-trust elements of the health and social services are entrusted with planning, overseeing and inspection functions, rather than with direct service provision.

- A care programming (a discharge plan) and care management (an assessment and purchasing plan) system is to be put into place for people with an assumed high level of need, including those discharged from hospital who require long-term intervention (see the section on care management in Chapter 4).

A very heated debate about the usefulness of each of these measures in achieving greater efficacy among specific services and the welfare system as a whole has just began, and we will need to wait for sometime for a balanced judgement to emerge. This extensive structural change also has far-reaching implications for a number of professional groups and for the relationship between service users, their relatives and professionals, which will be looked at in Chapters 5 and 7.

Other European countries too have changed some components of their welfare systems. In the early 1980s the Netherlands transferred health and social services in the community to not-for-profit foundations, retaining local government as a mere enabling body.[14] Italy has established a large network of cooperatives to provide social care. Health services are funded by insurance schemes in a number of European countries (Germany, the Netherlands, France).

In the early 1980s the principled choice was between the residual (targeting the few), institutional (targeting the whole population for certain aspects of living) or socialist (targeting the whole population for every aspect of living) models of welfare ideology. In the 1990s most European countries have moved more towards the residual approach, even though remnants of the institutional (universal) model remain at both the ideological and the service system level.

As suggested in the start of this chapter, people suffering from mental illness are usually also poor people, with all that comes with poverty: poor housing, debt, unemployment, poor physical health, the lack of opportunity to improve their lot in life (not ably education, contact with the right people in the right places, and sufficient disposable income), lack of participation in communal life, relative exclusion from leisure activities, poor personal appearance, and a low level of expectation and self-esteem. Thus changes in welfare policies – and the distribution mechanisms for welfare benefits – have a considerable impact on the everyday life of this group. This impact is compounded by the stigma attached to being a user of mental health services, social security and social services, in addition to the stigma attached to suffering from serious mental distress, and the impact of the suffering itself.

Emerging mental health policies

Pre-1980 policies

These policies were marked by four trends:

1. The introduction of comprehensive health and social welfare measures as universal entitlements in Europe led to a considerable expansion of mental health services. Both the number of hospitals and the number of beds increased, followed by an increase in the number of medical workers.[15]
2. The integration of psychiatry into medicine, according to the wishes of psychiatrists and nurses, and the belief of politicians and the general public in medicine. This was reflected in the establishment of psychiatric wards in general hospitals, perceived in the 1950s and 1960s as a more promising strategy than retaining large psychiatric hospitals.
3. An attempt to humanise psychiatric hospitals, expressed in greater attention to the in physical condition, the introduction of occupational therapy and sheltered work opportunities, as well as therapeutic communities in some hospitals.[16]
4. The adoption of an all-encompassing, but vague, community care ideology by politicians led to the development of services in the community, with hospitals forming the core of the psychiatric system.

The ideology and policies that followed throughout Europe were based on belief in the role that families and informal carers play in looking after disabled family members across the range of disabilities, ignoring the cost to unpaid carers in physical, emotional, financial and social terms. The fact that most of these carers were/are women highlights the gender implications of community care policies, further complicated by the fact that the majority of clients and paid workers are women too.[17]

As will be discussed in Chapter 4, resettlement of long-term residents of psychiatric hospitals into the community has *not* meant going back to their families, but living in non-family settings. However those known as 'the new long stay' and those hospitalised for short periods are likely to rely on their families either on a temporary or a permanent basis.

Pre-1980 mental health legislation

New mental health legislation was passed in Belgium (1969), Britain (1959), France (1968), Germany (mid 1970s) and Italy (1968 and 1978). With the exception of the Italian legislation, the rest focused in part on liberalising compulsory admission legislation and on tinkering with the structure of the service system (for example sectorisation in France).

The Italian Mental Treatment Law of 1978 (Law 180, as it is known) remains a unique act as it legislated for a complete restructuring of mental health services. The law dictated the following:[18]

1. The building of new hospitals would be stopped.
2. There would be no further admissions to psychiatric hospitals, but psychiatric wards of up to 15 beds per 200000 inhabitants would be made available in general hospitals.
3. Community mental health centres would be established to replace hospitals as the core providers of mental health services.
4. Compulsory admissions would be agreed by psychiatrists and city mayors.

With the exception of Italy, the pronounced shift towards care in the community for people suffering from serious mental illness was not accompanied by facilitating legislation. The reader interested in a comprehensive picture of pre-1980 mental health policies will find it in publications by Busfield, Goodwin, Louzoun, Mangen, and Ramon.[19]

Post-1980 policies

Dehospitalisation
The most striking departure with past tradition is the attempt to move away from relyiance on psychiatric hospitals as the core of

Table 1.1 Number of beds in 10 European countries, 1980 and 1990[20]

	1980	1990
Belgium	24 567	21 780
England & Wales	88 000	55 000
Finland	17 000	13 000
France	105 000	91 000
Western Germany	107 965	60 000
Greece	8149	6377
Italy	54 000	25 000
The Netherlands	26 730	26 200
Slovenia	1841	1594
Sweden	28 289	14 581

the mental health services in Western Europe. While Western European countries differ in the pace, range and depth of change, this change of direction can be detected in all countries (Table 1.1).

In some countries the change has taken the form of reducing psychiatric hospitals beds while increasing the number of beds in general hospitals, side by side with the introduction of community mental health centres (for example in Greece and Sweden). In two European countries (Italy and Britain), psychiatric hospitals have been closed but the number of psychiatric beds in general hospitals have been kept to a minimum. An increase in the number of secure provisions, while reducing all other bed facilities, has followed in Britain but not in Italy. Furthermore, while most hospital closures took place in Italy before 1985, the majority of British hospital closures date from 1985 (Figure 1.1).

Interestingly, policy solutions rarely include community asylum facilities *in any European country*. The facilities that do exist are described in Chapter 4.

Dehospitalisation was motivated by:

- A gradual reduction in the number of first admissions.
- A considerable decrease in the length of hospitalisation.
- Evidence demonstrating that people with long-term mental illness can live outside a hospital setting.

Emerging Policy Perspectives 27

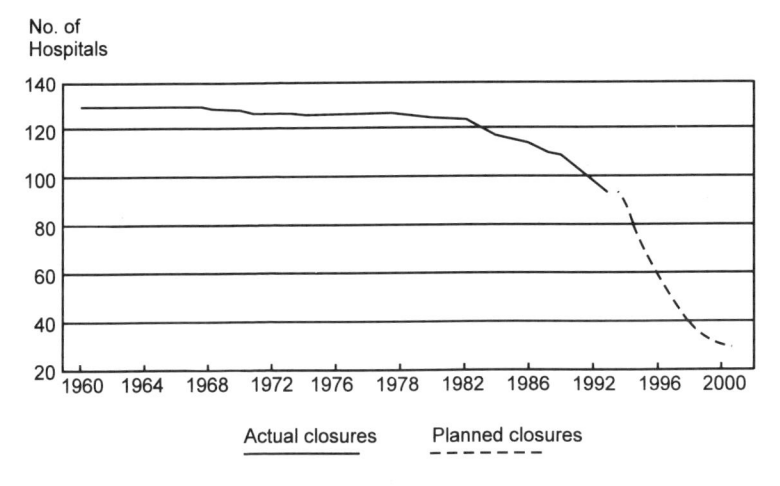

No. of Hospitals

[Graph showing hospital numbers declining from ~130 in 1960 to ~30 by 2000, with actual closures as solid line and planned closures as dashed line]

Actual closures ——————
Planned closures - - - - - -

Source: R. Hill, *Selected Issues in Mental Health: An Introductory Paper* (Sainsbury Mental Health Centre, November 1993).

Figure 1.1 Rate of English hospital closure, 1960–2000

- A critique concerning the using of psychiatric hospitals as the core of a mental health system.
- The spiralling costs of maintaining the old hospitals, and the cost of maintaining beds versus community facilities in general.
- The gradual development of alternative services outside hospitals.
- The impact of the North American example of hospital closure in the 1960s and 1970s, and later the impact of the Italian example of hospital closure in the 1970s and 1980s.
- The move to 'free market' economic policies and the ideological focus on reducing public expenditure.

The first two developments were interrelated, through changes in the focus of intervention (the introduction of the Open Door policy in the 1940s and 1950s, the introduction of psychotropic drugs in the 1960s, a greater focus on rehabilitation within the hospital and in the community from the 1950s onward, the availability of day services and out-patient clinics) and greater public tolerance since the Second World War, but especially since the 1960s. However these developments did not on their own lead to the policy shift, but merely enabled its acceptance.

The critique of the hospital as a social institution was more central to the formulation of the new policy. The critique came in four waves:[21] firstly from the United State, by humanist psychiatrists and sociologists; secondly from British psychiatrists, social workers and psychologists; thirdly from Italian psychiatrists, sociologists, nurses and social workers; and fourthly from service users in the United States in the 1970s and 1980s and Europe in the 1970s, 1980s and 1990s). Variations in their critiques in terms of conceptual and ideological underpinnings are outlined in Chapter 4.

The only group of major stakeholders not to criticise hospitals and hospitalisation were/are relatives (some of whom also act as unpaid carers), who are obviously keen on retaining a space that lets them off the hook both ideologically and practically. The overall message highlighted the damage created by hospitalisation, especially prolonged hospitalisation, to the rehabilitation prospects and self-identity of inpatients. While the debate continues on whether the harm done by hospitalisation constitutes primary or secondary damage, evidence of the success of rehabilitation programmes in the community makes it difficult to reject outright the advantages of community intervention as opposed to hospitalisation for most service users.[22]

The appeal to politicians from both the right and the left of the political spectrum is that greater freedom and improved chance of recovery combine with the promise of cost-cutting, turning community care into an almost irresistible proposition. The degree of irresistibility was and still is greater in the case of right-wing, 'free market' politicians as they are less committed than left-wing politicians to defending public sector services and their employees. Indeed Britain is a key example of a country with little or no professional push for dehospitalisation but with politicians adhering to a free market option that has gone much further along the road to dehospitalisation than in most other European countries.

Italy provides us with an example of a country pushed by a professional movement that has managed to capture enough public support to almost force the unwilling politicians to go ahead with a radical programme of hospital closure and deinstitutionalisation. France and Belgium exemplify the case of countries that lack professional pressure while having a well-developed public sector mental health system, ruled by politicians who either favour a public sector service system or are not that confident they can go ahead with a full-blown privatisation policy.

The Netherlands provides yet another case in point, of a country where most of the health services are delivered by insurance companies and foundations, which although in receipt of government sponsorship are nevertheless able to resist its policy control. While the central government seems keen on dehospitalisation, and has encouraged the development of user organisations and advocacy schemes partly for this purpose, it has not managed to dislodge the stronghold of its own creation of health delivery by insurance schemes.

It would therefore seem that the crucial factors in determining whether a member state is able to go ahead with a dehospitalisation programme depends on the combined effect of the motivations of its mental health professionals, its politicians, and the system of health and social care delivery.

A further central factor is how the health delivery system is funded, and which basic units are being funded. If beds or a hospital are the funded unit, it is much more difficult to achieve dehospitalisation than if the funded unit is a health district's mental health services.

The ease of transfer of funding within the same service and across services is also of great importance, as beds are notoriously expensive and can absorb all available funding if the transfer is not secured. Thus in Britain and Italy the much smaller number of beds available in 1994 continue to absorb 91 per cent and 75 per cent, respectively, of the health budget for mental health services, leaving community services with a very small share of the financial cake.[23] The planning of dehospitalisation depends not only on funding mechanisms, but even more on whether the aim of the exercise is to achieve dehospitalisation or *deinstitutionalisation*.

Deinstitutionalisation

Although all of the countries that have opted for dehospitalisation have claimed to be aiming at deinstitutionalisation, it is possible to detect whether this was the case or not by investigating the stated final objectives of the policy, and the types of alternatives to hospitals that have been encouraged by a government.

In principle, deinstitutionalisation is about ensuring that people suffering from serious mental breakdown or a serious permanent mental illness will be cared for in non-hospital settings, and supported in leading as ordinary a life as possible. Thus deinstitutionalisation is about actively preventing hospitalisation and ensuring community support for people with a serious mental illness.

While the first phase of the US programme – namely the establishment of community mental health centres in the 1960s – was an attempt to provide an alternative structure to outpatient clinics and could also be seen as a partial attempt to prevent admissions,[24] it was less focused on enabling continued care clients to live in the community. The massive wave of hospital closures in the late 1960s and 1970s provided this group with the basic necessities in the form of accommodation, income and day centre facilities. These were seen as sufficient to ensure rehabilitation in the community. Little attention was focused on *presence in the community, competence beyond self-care, and community participation*. Furthermore it was found that continued care clients were receiving little benefit from community mental health centres, and that not much had changed, apart from the introduction of some more assertive out-reach programmes.

Hospitals closure was not utilised in the US case as an opportunity to change the system, the attitudes or the skills of providers and purchasers, nor to increase the involvement of the lay community. I would argue that this was the case because the aim of the government, and a number of professionals, was not to reach beyond dehospitalisation. The latter was a finite objective for a cost-cutting exercise, as demonstrated by cuts in the budgets of community mental health centres a few years later.

The oscillation between dehospitalisation and deinstitutionalisation can be seen in a number of European countries, such as France, Spain and Sweden.[25] The on-going difficulty of recognising non-medical initiatives in the community as an integral part of the mental health system in Germany is highlighted by the exclusion of such interventions from the package of services that are reimbursed by insurance companies, while hospitalisation is recognised as a remunerable expense. Community living and preventative initiatives have therefore been slower to emerge and have to struggle continuously for their financial survival. The Dutch example mentioned above illustrates further the stranglehoold insurance schemes seem to have in securing the continuation of the more traditional ways of approaching mental health services.

The US experience has illustrated that profits can be made in nursing homes and closed secure units, besides hospitals. Ordinary services in the community may provide the members of private Italian health care cooperatives with enough to live on, but not to earn the high profit margins that a large company would expect.

In most Western European countries deinstitutionalisation is happening side by side with dehospitalisation, often without a government policy that favours deinstitutionalisation but through the use of channels opened by government policies aimed at mixed economies of care and mixed sectors of services. Portugal presents the only case in Western Europe of a government actively attempting to deter deinstitutionalisation.[26] The logic behind this decision is straightforward. If mental illness is a disease like any other disease then it should be treated in a medical setting. Hospitals are a medical setting par excellence; therefore hospitals are the best location for mental health services. Thus the Portugese decision highlights the inherent tension between continuing adherence to the medical model of mental illness and the alternative model where recognition of the difference between mental illness and other illnesses is paramount. It also pinpoints that unless this difference is accepted in full, deinstitutionalisation policies are not going to be made or followed through.

Lest we forget what a fully hospital-based system looks like, Eastern Europe, and in particular the CIS countries, remind us. Let us look at two emblematic examples.

The Kashenko hospital in Moscow has 5000 inpatients (2000 less than its 7000 official capacity) and 5000 staff, mostly unqualified nurses. It has a vast space at its disposal, a number of occupational therapy workshops, lots of crumbling buildings and an imposing management block (also in dire need of repair). Upon admission, patients are stripped and washed with disinfectant. Wards contain up to 40 beds, with no private space. They are spacious and very cold, as heating is expensive and erratic. There are cracks in the walls and floors, the sanitation is poor and all wards – and workshops – are locked. Most of the menial work required in the hospital is carried out by the patients. Staff who leave are not replaced, but their (very small) salaries are added to the salaries of the remaining staff to entice them to stay. The only recent innovation is provided by members of the Methodist Church, who visit once a week on a befriending scheme, which seems to consist of a religious session. Yet its director considers that the residents will fare worse outside the hospital in the current economic and social conditions. He is right, as the existing welfare and psychiatric services are unable to meet the needs of much less institutionalised people, let alone the more institutionalised. Does this mean that nothing can be done as long as the current conditions prevail, apart from preserving the hospital-based system as it is?

A possible alternative has been adopted during the prolonged process of hospital closure in Italy. There the focus was on *changing the institution from within*, prior to any attempt to move people to the outside world. The logic behind this policy was that institutionalisation itself constitutes a prolonged way of living and internalised beliefs and identities on the part of both residents and staff, which in turn has been imposed on them by the community, but also projected from the hospital onto the community. Therefore attempting to change this state of affairs requires the gradual deinstitutionalisation of those who have suffered most from it, mainly residents and staff. The process itself consists of involving residents not only in the running of the hospital, but also in decision making and introducing a style of living that is more similar to that existing outside. This includes getting to know the community and the community becoming involved in activities inside the hospital. Successful Italian experiences highlight that:[27]

- hospitals can become fully open a short while after commencement of the transformation process;
- there are people in the community who are able and willing to contribute to the lives of the patients;
- staff can change their attitudes and skills to benefit themselves and the residents;
- residents can lead a more normal life (with support) and enjoy it, and most of them can become producers of social and material goods.

The Kashenko hospital is larger than most European villages, and has more financial and human resources available to it than most Russian villages, all of which could be put into transforming the institution into a self-regulating and productive community. For that to happen, however, a number of necessary and sufficient conditions need to be met, including:

- The leadership within the hospital should be ready to experiment, to let go of its highly authoritarian power and privileges. It should be committed to an alternative vision of mental distress, the people suffering from it, and mental health services.
- A state of preparedness at the regional level of the health services and the municipality level.
- Support from professional organisations and voluntary organisations.
- Ongoing advice, consultation and modelling by leaders of similar initiatives abroad.
- Such advice should include advice on the financial aspects of the internal transfer of resources, on making connections with the outside world, and on working with staff and residents.

The second emblematic Eastern European example is Hungary, where there are fewer large psychiatric hospitals but many units in general hospitals. There have about 100 inpatients, including children, adolescents, and alcohol and drug abusers side by side with people experiencing their first mental distress crisis. Wards usually have up to 50 people and contain beds, dining areas and sometimes a recreation area. Spotlessly clean, they smell of strong disinfectant; and the pervading near silence is like that preceeding or following a storm. There are very few nurses, few experienced psychiatrists or psychologists, and no social workers or trained occupational therapists.

Most of the professionals' time is taken up by assessments and prescriptions, and restraining alcoholics and drug addicts. Many discharged patients repeatedly return to hospital as there is nowhere else for them to go. Experienced psychiatrists and psychologists tend to work in outpatient clinics, teach at a university (preferably a private one), and by now may also be attempting to establish a private practice. Psychiatric wards in general hospitals have become dumping grounds for beginners and those who have failed to succeed elsewhere.

The presence of so many wards for children and adolescents is a legacy of the conviction that collective living is better then family living and that big is beautiful, which was part and parcel of the communist ideology and one of its means of control. Usually the children's wards are better furnished and decorated then adult wards. Nevertheless they too highlight the belief in total institutions as a positive social asset. Such a belief was once present in the West too, but was discarded soon after the Second World War following revelations of the slow development and emotional deprivation that were manifest in institutionalised children.

Not unlike his Russian colleague, the Hungarian psychiatrist who directs the unit I visited just outside Budapest (though the one in Pecs is smaller) felt that his unit was providing a much needed respite and cure space that was not available outside the hospital. A dedicated man who was aware that he had been abandoned by more experienced colleagues for financial and professional reasons, he was much less authoritarian than his Russian colleague (but then he was not the director of an institution with 10 000 people!) He lamented the fact that a lack of resources had led to the closure of the only room to offer occupational therapy. He seemed unaware of the connection between the lack of any activity on the ward for the relatively young and robust alcoholics and the degree of mayhem they created from time to time. Likewise he did not suggest that patients could effectively run these activities, which require very little staff supervision. He had no views on the type of services he would like to see established outside the hospital, but instead wanted to have more beds, more staff and more activities inside the hospital.

At the other end of the Hungarian spectrum, there is a lot of interest in individual and group psychotherapy, which was espoused during the communist regime in some places and is currently being reasserted by psychiatrists and psychologists who believe in its superiority over a somatic approach to mental illness.

The Hungarian director was right in some way, although it is possible to work with alcoholics more successfully outside a hospital unit then inside it. Detoxification does not require hospitalisation, even though it does initially require a residential setting. As AA has successfully demonstrated, it requires a non-psychotherapeutic group that also offers ongoing support outside the group. Individuals may benefit from individual and group psychotherapy, or from replacement medication in the case of drug abuse, but what they do not need is hospitalisation. The Hungarian director director could have encouraged the development of an AA movement in his unit and short-term respite and crisis facilities attached to primary health care centres; he could have attached an outpatient consultation service to primary care instead of retaining it in the hospital, and established foster families for most of the children and adolescents in the psychiatric ward.

Certain conditions will be necessary to enable change to take place, the most important of which in the Hungarian case would be a change in attitude among psychiatrists, as Hungary has a voluntary sector in the making, an AA-like tradition, and family consultation centres. Indeed one of the most positive experiences I had in Hungary was a visit to a group meeting of Hungarian and Gypsy men suffering from alcohol abuse (some of their wives and children were also present) in a small town near the border with Serbia.

With dehospitalisation and deinstitutionalisation come policies concerning *reprovision*.[28] These usually reflect whether dehospitalisation or deinstitutionalisation was intended, whether cost-cutting or cost-effectiveness was the government's leading motive, whether professional planners or professionals in mental health had the main say, whether health or social care was the priority, whether any attention was paid to processes and not only to outcomes, and whether or not the main stakeholders had a say. Reprovision includes solutions to issues such as housing, day activities, income, access to communal services and continuous clinical supervision. The specific solution adopted depends on the particular viewpoint adhered to, and the mechanisms by which resources are redistributed. Only in the British case has a closure and reprovision policy led to the creation of a number of small, closed ('secure') units for people defined as having challenging behaviour.

At the local level reprovision can be imaginative or unimaginative within the same budget and with the same distributary mechanisms, as solutions depend not only on ideological positions or financial resources, but on the individuals and teams entrusted with the job, their degree of interest and their ability to involve others. Specific examples of reprovision, and of the processes of hospital closure and resettlement in the community, are discussed in Chapter 4.

Funding and costs

Mental health services are usually funded by health authorities or insurance companies. Increasingly social services pay for the social care component, either by providing such care directly or by financing the private sector.

To facilitate hospital closure, the British government has provided a special 'dowry' for each long-stay resident of a psychiatric hospital transferred to the outside, usually to the local authority. Dowries have varied from £11 000 to £20 000, and have proved very popular.

A second British measure aimed at fostering innovation in working with continued care clients in the community is the Mental Health Specific Grant scheme, which has been in operation since 1991. Local authorities are provided with sums of up to £100 000 plus a third more is added by the local authority to fund specific projects. The health authorities have to approve each project, which is usually carried out by a social services team or a not-for-profit organisation. Again, these grants have proved very popular and out of 120 authorities, 110 have applied for them. Projects set up with this funding range from resource centres, advocacy schemes, special support occasional workers, to care management teams. It is unclear what will happen when the grants come to an end, as the scheme was only intended to be short term. This uncertainty has led to reduced commitment among workers on these schemes.

In Italy no special funding schemes were set up to facilitate hospital closures, but it was possible for the services transferred from the hospital to the community to retain their previous budgets, provided the director was politically astute.

One of the main attractions of dehospitalisation and deinstitutionalisation has been the claim that it will cost less than hospitalisation. *Cost measurement* has become an important issue, as initial calculations comparing hospital versus community services did not take into account indirect costs, such as the use of services in the community other than health services. Furthermore, to be useful, costs have to be looked at from the perspective of *cost effectiveness*, that is, whether the objectives for which the money is spent are achieved in the more or the less expensive service.[29] A related issue is whether costs increase or decrease over time for a person remaining in the same environment.

There are relatively few detailed studies on this subject, and even fewer in Europe. O'Donoll has looked at a mixture of studies carried out in the United States, Canada, Australia and the UK, plus one German study, all focusing on continued care clients.[30] Outcomes and costs of hospital-based alternatives to hospitalisation (for example day hospital and hospital hostel) were compared. He concluded that we lack sufficient evidence as to the efficacy of community care for this group, even though comprehensive programmes of support in the community have demonstrated greater efficacy than inpatient admission. His caution came out of the small number of such studies and the variety of individuals – and their needs – that any cost-effectiveness analysis must take into account.

Knapp and his colleagues at Kent University, and now at the Institute of Psychiatry in London, have carried out most of the British work on the cost of reprovision.[31] Table 1.2 illustrates the distribution of costs of reprovision, and the average cost to the community versus the hospital per week.

Knapp *et al.* looked at outcomes measures (that is, effectiveness of the reprovision programmes) and suggested that 'The comprehensive costs of the community care packages, based on the best economic principles of long-run marginal opportunity costing, were in fact found to be lower than the full costs of inpatient hospitalisation, even after adjustment for the tendency of projects to take clients who were less dependent than the hospital average' (ibid., p. 324).

A different type of costing is looked at when a specific type of intervention, such as a new medication, is considered in comparison with similar interventions. For example Davies and Drummond recently investigated the costs and benefits of Clozapine therapy for people judged to be otherwise 'treatment-resistant'.[32] They were interested in the efficacy of the new drug in terms of both symptom reduction and side effects, its financial cost, how many years it would add to people's lives, and whether their lives would be free of disability or with only mild disability. The research was conducted by asking UK specialists

Table 1.2 Community care costs by place of residence for people with mental health problems (per cent)

Community care component	Percentage of total package cost by place of residence in the community[1]							
	Resid.	Host.	Sgh	Usgh	Indep.	Fost.	Supp.	All places
Accommodation and living expenses[2]	66	71	68	42	62	60	57	61
Project overheads[3]	0	4	6	12	7	0	11	6
General practitioner	0	0	0	1	0	0	1	0
Day activity services	12	16	14	21	22	31	19	17
Education	0	1	0	1	3	3	1	0
Inpatient hospital	15	1	6	1	0	0	0	3
Out-and day patient hospital	0	2	2	1	0	0	0	1
Community health care[4]	6	2	3	5	1	1	2	3
Community social care	0	2	2	17	4	3	6	10
Other[5]	0	0	0	0	0	0	0	0
Total (%)	100	100	100	100	100	100	100	100
Sample size	11	52	13	40	6	5	3	130
Community cost[6]	374	269	325	243	222	260	181	271
Hospital cost[6]	386	330	380	363	362	354	359	354

Notes:
1. Accommodation codes are: Resid. = residential home; Host. = hostel; Sgh = staffed group home; Usgh = unstaffed group home; Indep. = independent accommodation; Fost. = adult fostering; Supp. = supported lodgings.
2. Includes staff costs where staff are employed solely at the place of residence and are included in the accommodation budget.
3. Inclusions vary from project to project, usually covering some immediate managerial support and some peripatetic staff support.
4. Includes community nursing, medical practitioners not attached to hospital or family practices, miscellaneous community health paramedic services (chiropody, dietary services, incontinence service, and so on).
5. Includes police, travel not covered elsewhere and miscellaneous services.
6. Costs expressed in pounds at 1986–87 price levels per client per week.

Source: M. Knapp *et al., Care in the Community: Challenge and Demonstration* (Canterbury: Personal Social Services Research Unit, University of Kent, 1992), p. 316.

to express their view in relation to a clinical decision tree that listed the probabilities of patients achieving different outcomes due to the application of different drugs. The probabilities were derived from a US sample of 47 patients. On the basis of this procedure the researchers concluded that 'For the patients themselves clozapine would lead to a net gain of 5.87 years of life with no disability or only mild disability. The base case analysis showed that the direct costs of using clozapine were £91 less per annum than the standard neuroleptic therapy'.[33] This method of research and the decisions based on it raise a number of doubts, chiefly whether the comparison was one of like-with-like, and whether the comparison took real life differences sufficiently into account.

Post-1980 legislation

A similar wave to the one that took place mainly in the 1960s occurred in the 1980s. New and amended acts were passed in Britain, Denmark, Greece, Ireland, Luxembourg, Spain and Sweden. A clear division emerges, in that the British, Irish and Spanish legislations focused on patients' rights and procedures for compulsory admission, whereas the others focused more on restructuring the service system by shifting services to the community and psychiatric hospitalisation to general hospitals.

The British 1983 amendments to the 1959 Mental Health Act introduced a small number of significant changes. First, a new body was created – the Mental Health Act Commission, whose task is to oversee the procedure of compulsory admissions and the way detained patients are treated. The Commission is divided into two in England and Wales, with a separate Commission in Scotland. Commissioners are nominated by the secretary of state for Health on a part-time basis, and are either mental health professionals or representatives of the community health councils (an advisory body). No users or their relatives can be members of the Commission, and no representative of users' or relatives' organisations is included. Headed by lawyers, the Commission has undertaken inspection visits and made recommendations for changes to the institutions visited, talked to detained patients, and made recommendations to the minister of health, including proposals for new legislation and inquiry committees when relevant.[34]

While an important tool in principle, the Commission's mandate does not allow it to look at most issues of professional intervention that are not focused on procedural legal processes, and these remain largely unaccountable. Legally individuals can sue named professionals involved in compulsory admission and detention (for example psychiatrists, social workers and nurses). Apart from cases of maltreatment in special hospitals (discussed in Chapter 4) this right has not been exercised to date.

Second, some types of intervention can be categorised by the Commission as at times leading to irreversible harm to the person thus treated. In such a case the patient has to provide his/her informed consent, and the independent view of a psychiatrist who is not from the same health authority is required in addition to the recommendation of the psychiatrist in charge. The Commission has agreed that hormonal treatment and psychosurgery constitute such interventions. Since 1991 the commission has been divided over the question of electroconvulsive therapy (ECT) and has been unable to reach a decision.

This change in legislation is of considerable importance in acknowledging that intervention is not only helpful, but can also be harmful in some circumstances, and that some interventions are potentially more harmful than others. It is a landmark in that it requires professionals to rethink clinical decisions, seek formal advice, take account of whether or not the patient has agreed to the treatment and inform the patient about the different effects of the intervention; and in that the professional may be refused permission to carry out the intervention if overruled by the independent psychiatrist.

Despite outstanding issues such as how to ensure that patients are adequately informed and not under undue pressure to give their consent, and the lack of involvement of any other professional or lay figures as originally proposed in 1978, this development paves the way for a qualitatively different type of professional accountability from those exercised presently in Europe.

Third, guardianship orders were introduced whereby users have to frequent specific locations, live at a specified address and be under the general supervision of a nominated key worker, usually a local authority social worker. Although guardianship previously existed in British legislation, it was not in use. Its reintroduction opened the legal way to the possibility of *community supervision orders* (a proposal that will be looked at in Chapter 4), which exist in Canada and some parts of the United States (for example Virginia and North Carolina).

Guardianship also exists in Italian law for detained patients discharged from a psychiatric prison. However this guardianship is exercised by a multidisciplinary mental health team, and not by one professional. Likewise the exact conditions are not specified, and are decided by a judge in consultation with the patient and the service in each case.

Fourth, a mandatory aftercare planning order has been put into place (Section 117) for people discharged after being compulsorily admitted. This amounts to a meeting of the professionals involved with the patient and relatives (if they are involved) to plan the discharge and its aftermath. It does not cover the implementation of the decisions taken in the planning meeting, or provision of the resources necessary for such an implementation.

Fifth, the legal involvement of social workers in the process of decision making concerning compulsory admission dates from 1959. The 1983 legislation strengthened this legal position by establishing the status of an Approved Social Worker (ASW) and by requiring specific training to be successfully completed for this purpose by the holders of this title. At present 60 training days are required initially, with some updating days later on.

The implications of this change to the roles of social workers and their reactions to this development are looked at in Chapter 7. At this stage it is important to note that Britain continues to be the only European country that has given its social workers such responsibility, which includes recognising the importance of the psychosocial perspective in crucial mental health decision making, such as compulsory admission. The reader interested in learning more about how this change works in practice is advised to read Barnes *et al.*'s study of the activities of ASWs in 43 local authorities.[35]

None of the other new structures (outlined in Chapter 4) come out of mental health policies, but of policies related to the organisation, and structures and modes of delivery of health and social care in European societies. At times these can have a crucial effect on mental health services, as in:

42 Mental Health in Europe

- the German case of not recognising social care as a reimbursed expense;
- legislation that holds relatives formally responsible for the care of disabled family members (Germany);
- decreeing the use of non-public-sector services (Britain's latest legislation on community care stipulates that local authorities have to use 85 per cent of the community care grant on private provisions);
- freezing new posts in public services (enforced in Italy for the last five years);
- a disproportionate continuous spending on beds rather then on community services in all European countries;
- limitations on the earnings allowed without loss of disability benefits (which act as a disincentive to employment for many people with disabilities in most European countries);
- not being allowed to work once a person is registered as disabled (CIS and other East European countries);
- separation of the providers and purchasers of all public sector services (in Britain since April 1993);
- the introduction of care programming and care management for all community care services (Britain, the Netherlands), which will be looked at in Chapter 4.

Thus both direct mental health policies and indirect welfare policies influence the objectives of mental health services, their activities, and their style of operation. The implications of the major policies for users, carers and workers, as well as for service structures, will be examined in Chapters 4, 5 and 6. In part, Chapter 7 will reflect reactions to the policies and the ways in which they have been implemented.

Summary

During the 1980s and 1990s we have witnessed considerable changes in the social context in which mental health policies are decided upon and implemented. A fundamental shift in mental health policies has taken place, and this has led to an array of structural changes in the wider (welfare) and narrower (mental health) service systems throughout Europe, ending some structures and beginning some new ones. The unevenness of the rate and depth of change in each country depends on the specific interactions between the changes in the context and the influence of major stakeholders of mental health systems (politicians, professionals, users and relatives, the media). The rest of this book looks at the major interpretations, applications and implications of the policies portrayed above to European mental health systems and their stakeholders.

2
Conceptual Innovations

The concepts of dehospitalisation, deinstitutionalisation and demarginalisation that underlie the policies outlined in Chapter 1 were initially developed in the United States and Western Europe during the 1960s. New concepts and theoretical frameworks that have emerged since the beginning of the 1980s in the countries discussed below include:

- continued care clients;
- normalisation and social role valorisation;
- deconstruction of the classical psychiatric diagnostic system (schizophrenia, expressed emotions, challenging behaviour, accepting voices);
- sexual abuse as an everyday phenomenon;
- the emergence of new stakeholders: users and relatives as reactive and proactive actors.

Continued care clients

The rediscovery of this group as worthy of social, political and professional attention first took off during the 1960s and 1970s in Italy and Switzerland, France, Germany, the Netherlands and the United States, arriving in Britain in the middle of the 1980s.[1] It meant firstly the rediscovery of the group as having the potential to lead a non-institutionalised life, albeit with continuous support. This was based on the discovery of their qualities as people, to include *abilities* and not only disabilities, diagnosis and prognosis, regardless of whether they resided in psychiatric institutions or outside them. It took place as the combined result of the following developments:

- rehabilitation programmes in the United States and Britain;[2]
- the specific process of hospital closure in Italy, which enabled these people to reemerge as human beings with distinct individualised features;[3]

- the long-term follow-up of people diagnosed as suffering from schizophrenia in Switzerland;[4]
- social psychiatric projects in France and Germany;
- advocacy projects in the Netherlands;
- the more recent explicit impact of the normalisation approach.

Conceptually this development relates to the demarginalisation movement that took place in Europe during the 1960s and 1970s. This has enabled us to respect people with a recognised disability as people – even when, and/or because, they have been segregated and largely invisible for a long period – as part of the impact of the new social movements[5]. The shift took place at a time when a number of minorities were gaining a more prominent and positive social place (for example women and young people), while other minorities were continuing to struggle for such acceptance (for example black people and gay people).

The ambiguities concerning the social acceptability of a hitherto undesirable minority group have been highlighted on more than one level. First, the term continued care client denotes an on-going recipient of mental health services who is in need of their support. Thus doubt is cast on the likelihood of a long-lasting recovery, a measure of continuing disability is assumed and a suspended identity is attributed to individual members of this group. Yet this precarious identity was sufficient to allow them move out of the asylum and be redefined as *deserving* social support in the community.

As Christine McCourt Perring has illustrated,[6] one way of handling this new ambiguous identity is of viewing users as children who will not grow up. Mini-institutions are another way of rendering them *socially invisible*, even if they are *physically visible*.

Second, the demonisation of continued care clients, explored below, is associated with terms such as 'persistently and severely mentally ill'. This implies that most continued care clients are likely to erupt into violent and unpredictable behaviour that may endanger all of us at any time, thus making us doubt their ability to live amongst us.

Third, at the other end of the conceptual and attitudinal spectrum, the disability movement claims that disability is a problem because of the way so-called non-disabled people approach those defined as disabled, and not because of the constraints introduced by the disability itself.[7] Taking their cue from the deviancy approach, its protagonists argue forcefully that left to themselves people with a physical disability do not see themselves as inferior to other people; if anything they view themselves as superior to non-disabled people as a result of having to struggle to overcome their specific physical constraints, thus gaining in sensitivity and survival skills, or in having to counteract daily the social stigma attached to them.

All of these issues are put into a sharper focus in relation to people suffering from mental distress. Are they disabled? Are they temporarily so? Does their disability relate to all of their being, or only to some specified aspects? Can they make decisions for themselves? Is their decision-making ability impaired in some aspects but not others? Is it the effect of the intervention that is impairing their decision making? (See the debate on the impact of medication in Chapter 4.)

Continued care clients therefore are likely to continue to live with a 'threatened identity', a term coined by Glenys Breakwell[8] in her analysis of a variety of marginal identities of people who transgress specific social boundaries, either intentionally or unintentionally (for example people who change their sex, unemployed people, members of ethnic minorities). They respond to the internal and/or external threat by developing a number of interpsychic, interpersonal and intergroup coping strategies, the choice of which depends on the nature of the threat, its social context, and their identity structure and cognitive resources. Table 2.1 presents the main coping strategies available to people in a state of threatened identity.

How we construct the fragile identity of reemergent members of our society will also determine whether they can utilise more constructive coping strategies and eventually rebuild a less threatened identity.

Elsewhere I have suggested that the act of leaving a hospital can be used to signify a positive reentry, if we so choose socially.[9] Yet most service users I have talked to about this issue have found leaving to be a negative experience. The few who experienced leaving in positive terms saw it as a raft on an otherwise turbulent sea.

The initial entry into the 'moral career of the mental patient', to use Goffman's concept[10] (that is, hospital admission), can also be

Table 2.1 Coping strategies when facing a threat to self-identity

Interpsychic	Interpersonal	Intergroup
Modification through assimilation:		
1. Deflection	Isolation	Membership
2. Acceptance	Negativism	Group support
Modification through evaluation:	Passing	Group action
1. Reevaluation of current identity	Compliance	
2. Reevaluation of prospective identity		

Source: G. Breakwell, *Coping with Threatened Identities* (London, Methuen, 1986), pp. 80, 108, 129.

treated with explicit attention to its symbolic meaning, by minimising the disruption to ordinary living, the reinterpretation of the past and the invention of a *reversible* future. Retreat facilities in the community provide one example of this approach.

With the rediscovery of the continued care client came the inevitable critique of past practices, together with shame, blame, guilt, defensiveness and a desire for reparation; all of which are uncomfortable to live with for all of us, but especially for those who have worked in the hospitals.[11]

However the hedging form which the rediscovery took has perhaps prevented us from leading to a reconsideration of the value of psychiatric diagnosis on its own, and of our understanding of the nature of mental illness. Thus, at most, the rediscovery of the continued care client turned a fully closed door into a half-open one.

The significance of the identity of the rediscoverer

In Britain it was the government that was the main discoverer of the continued care client; as was the case in the Netherlands, aided by service user groups. In Italy, Germany and France the discovery was made by a minority of mental health professionals. This is not to say that other sectors have not made the rediscovery too, but that they made it in a less prominent way.

The identity of the rediscoverer is significant in terms of the likely impact of the rediscovery and the emphasis put on it. Thus the rediscovery of the continued care client by the British government was motivated by the knowledge that a hospital closure cannot take place without the resettlement of its long-stay users. It has also led to a much greater targeting of this group as eligible for care management (see Chapter 4) and a reduction in the traditional neglect of this group by politicians and professionals. At the same time it seems to mean a sanctioned neglect of the less distressed and vulnerable, and a neglect of work that could prevent a number of people from becoming continued care clients in the first place.

User participation has been recently encouraged by the British government through the National Mental Health Task Force (described in Chapter 1). One of the government's motives for this initiative was to change professional performance and attitudes through pressure from users. Likewise, in the Netherlands the rediscovery was used by the government as a tool to develop a potential pressure group against the private insurance companies that control the hospital sector, and which refuse to close such institutions. Pressure groups have had a beneficial impact in creating an elaborate advocacy scheme and giving users a voice in planning, as well as in improving living conditions in hospitals. However they have not been able to exert sufficient pressure to have psychiatric hospitals closed or an alternative conceptual framework created.

The rediscovery of continued care clients by professionals in Italy indeed meant a radical shift in the way the minority who pioneered the reform approached mental distress and the people who suffer from it, leading to their becoming community organisers and educators first, and therapist or psychiatrist second.

Negative responses to the rediscovery

Relatives and a growing number of prominent professionals who nowaday prefer to use the term 'severely and persistently mentally ill' are also active in the field of psychiatric rehabilitation.[12] When asked why they use this rather derogatory term, the reply is that it is more accurate and realistic than other terms, and it does not attempt to gloss over the disability and disease inherent in the situation. It correlates closely with the view that continued care clients have a poor prognosis, cannot lead an ordinary life without very meticulous control and attention, and present a permanent high risk.[13]

The subcategory 'the new long stay' (the 'old long stay' being the majority of resettled ex-patients) has captured the imagination of those who coined the concept of the severely mentally ill.[14] The new long stay are relatively young people, often diagnosed as schizophrenic, and sometimes also associated with substance abuse, with multiple admissions that become progressively longer. They are much less compliant than the old long stay and therefore do not take medication regularly or are seen as 'not responding to medication'. They are more articulate and vocal, and at times more assertive/aggressive than the old long stay. They have disrupted family relationships but nevertheless return frequently to the family home. There are more men than women among this group, and a much higher proportion than previously are members of specific ethnic minorities.

It is this group, exposing as it does the limitations of the usefulness of psychiatry in both its caring and controlling functions, that has become the focus of a *demonisation* campaign in the United States and in Britain, *but nowhere else* (at least for the time being).

Demonisation takes a number of forms, such as a consistent portrayal of everyone in the group as dangerous, violent and unpredictable, laced with pity or calling for such people to be locked up 'for their own good' as well as for the safety of others. For example, under the headline 'Free to kill in the community' (*Daily Mail*, 2 July 1993), Mr D. Williams – described as 'chief reporter' – outlines five cases of people being killed by diagnosed sufferers of mental illness. In a paragraph in which he describes one such brutal killing, he goes on to say that 250 000 people suffer from symptoms of schizophrenia in Britain, thus implying that each of the 250 000 is likely to commit a murder. To the best of our knowledge on this subject, this is far from being the case. Most murders in our society are committed by people who have not been diagnosed as suffering from mental illness prior to the specific event. While statistically there is a greater likelihood that people will commit murder when actively mentally ill than people who do not suffer from schizophrenia, the main risk is that they will harm themselves rather than others.[15]

In an article by Ms Wallace, chief executive of Sane (Schizophrenia, A National Emergency), assures us that she had the courage to describe 'what was happening in Italy and America, where the closure of hospitals has been accelerated. As a result, thousands of sick, abandoned people crowded the railway stations and streets'. I have visited different cities in Italy for the last fourteen years, including major cities such as Rome, Milan, Turin and Naples. I have never seen thousands, or even hundreds, or tens, of sick or dispossessed people crowding train stations in any one of these cities, let alone thousands of mentally ill people. I have seen homeless people in the United States and Britain, some of whom are suffering from mental illness, either becoming mentally ill after drifting into homelessness or already mentally ill and becoming homeless due to government policies. The leap from this state of affairs, which I would join in condemning, to the insinuation that most ex-patients in Italy, the United States and Britain are murderers in waiting is preposterous. The fact that her words were published, that Ms Wallace is allowed to continue with her insinuations, is a reflection of the readiness of the media to use demonisation as a way of selling news and newspapers.

To demonise means to attribute drastically negative qualities to people who do not usually demonstrate such behaviour, or as Cohen has suggested, they are the new 'folk devils'.[16] Demonisation is not a too strong a term to use when:

- an undifferentiating campaign is taking place, when a relatives' and psychiatrists' organisation feels justified in putting posters in railway stations that depict such people as killers;[17]
- the overall positive statistics about the outcomes of planned resettlement do not figure in any of the media coverage, but transgression by one person known to be mentally ill becomes front page news;
- representatives of the organisation spearheading the demonisation are regular contributors in the media; users opposing this campaign are not;
- the first case of a mass killing in Britain, committed by a person not known to have suffered from mental illness, was greeted with a headline that had no backing whatsoever in the history of psychiatry: 'matricide points to schizophrenia';[18]

Conceptual Innovations 51

- the backers of the defaming organisation call for a halt to hospital closure and for the introduction of legal controlling measures that will force more people to spend more time in hospital and be on a formal register of the 'dangerously mentally ill';
- in the wake of North American legislation, the British government introduced a register of such people by health authorities (April 1994), and is considering proposals for a community supervision order where not taking medication will be a sufficient reason for hospitalisation, on the assumption that a mental deterioration is bound to happen to anyone in this category who stops taking medication. Neither the government nor the spearheading organisation have taken any notice of the rejection of community treatment orders by a House of Commons Select Health Committee in July 1993 as neither useful nor desirable.

Indeed demonisation is the process by which a group of people are attributed generalised qualities that fit the stereotyped judgement upon which demonisation is based, rather than allowing them to be as different from each other as most people are, and to have both positive and negative qualities. Thus demonisation is achieving the opposite of that achieved by the rediscovery of the continued care client as a human being. It would be foolhardy to ignore the potential increase in risk of either self-harm or harm to others that has been associated with the new long-stay group. However, between taking account of such a risk and attempting to prevent it on the one hand, and demonising a large group of people on the other hand, there is a big gap. Those engaged in demonisation know that such an approach sells in the media, which is forever seeking the sensational, and attracts rich backers who are particularly frightened by elements likely to disrupt the social order that enables them to be rich. While people at the top are not necessarily cynical, they are ready to ignore facts and statistics, as well as to endanger the fragile balance of self-confidence and social acceptance of this group of people for the sake of measures already disproved as useful.

Demonisation appears to be a last-ditch move by psychiatrists who would rather force people into hospitals than examine where they have gone wrong, either conceptually and/or in terms of intervention methods, who are ready to distort facts and disregard research findings in the process.

As already mentioned, it is important to note that no similar development has taken place in Europe. Italy is of particular relevance here. Despite the fact that larger numbers of continued care clients are resettled in the community than in Britain, that there are fewer hospital beds in general hospitals and that fewer psychiatric hospitals remain, neither the media nor relatives have attempted to put this type of pressure on politicians. They must be all blind, as they have obviously not seen Ms Wallace's 'thousands of people abandoned in the railway stations'. In turn there is no sign that politicians are using potential risk as a way of changing the psychiatric system, or for political gain. This difference attests to the success of the Italian reform in fostering attitudinal change, and to the failure of its British counterpart to do so.

Normalisation and social role valorisation

Although developed in Denmark and Sweden in the late 1950s and in the United States during the 1960s and 1970s, the normalisation principle was acknowledged in Britain only from the beginning of the 1980s.[19] Neither the concept of normalisation nor that of social role valorisation are in use in Southern, Central or Eastern Europe, although their meaning has been adhered to in Italy from the beginning of the Italian psychiatric reform in the early 1960s.

Normalisation is a much clearer concept than community care (the global term used for the new policies) as it focuses on the right of people with any kind of disability (including mental distress) to an ordinary life, on the provision of opportunities for such a life and the removal of material and attitudinal obstacles to it.

Social role valorisation (SRV) – a term coined by Wolfensberger in 1983 in response to the critique of the principle of normalisation – concentrates specifically on the need of people to lead a *life valued by them and by the society of which they are members*. Wolfensberger has analysed the *devaluing* that has taken place in the lives of people with a disability, especially those in institutions.[20] His analysis is very similar to the one reached independently by the Italians. He focuses on symbolic devaluation, which is expressed in very concrete terms, such as:

- the location of places of intervention, and how they are architecturally structured;
- the language we use in talking to and about people with a disability;
- the please leave in the plural
- lack of opportunities experienced by people with disabilities to participate in valued ordinary spheres of activities and the cycle thus created of being unable to prove their ability, or improve their competencies, social image and standing.

Normalisation and social role valorisation represent a radical departure from the traditional illness approach to mental distress and from the inherent unclarity of community care by combining:

- preaching, criticising, analysing;
- putting into practice ways of perceiving people with serious disabilities as dignified individuals who each have something positive to offer others, and ways of enabling them to lead a dignified life.

The classical approach has been criticised as too white, middle class and male orientated,[21] as commanding conformity, and as overlooking the impact of people's disabilities on their functioning and social presentation. I do not think that these criticisms are inherent in the approach and represent only the view of some of its protagonists. Yet the lack of emphasis on group solidarity and the overemphasis on individualism is inherent. The latter deprives people with disabilities and those close to them of access to a major analytical tool and a way of being and working. A further missing link is the lack of serious attention to issues of self-risk and risk to others, despite the emergence of *gentle teaching*[22] as a promising conceptual and intervention alternative to the more coercive and controlling practices that still abound and those proposed for the future.

An intriguing critique has come from an application of Foucault's approach to the analysis of the historical treatment of both madness and sexuality in modern times to the normalisation approach. Rose and Adlam[23] have argued that the approach represses the right of people to express themselves through madness, as it concentrates on their non-mad part and encourages the dominance of this part at the exclusion of the mad aspect.

The approach has made many professionals uncomfortable and defensive, as it amounts to a judgement of their attitudes and work as often harmful to the users they serve. Other professionals have welcomed it as a timely correction to the condescending approach that has typified traditional work in all disciplines.

Its success to date has been more pronounced in people suffering from learning difficulties, the initial area in which SRV was developed. Yet there have also been notable successes in the area of mental distress – in enabling people to gain dignity and respect, in learning to live with the impact of mental distress yet exploring to the full their other qualities, and in fostering opportunities for solidarity.[24]

Deconstruction of the classical psychiatric diagnostic system

The process of deconstructing traditional psychiatric concepts has taken place throughout the relatively short history of Western psychiatry. It was particularly in evidence in the 1960s and 1970s around the application of the concept of total institutions and generalised deviancy, and in the critique advanced by the different branches of the antipsychiatry movement.[25] These approaches continued to develop in the 1980s, branching out on issues of control, gender and ethnicity. Psychoanalytical approaches, family therapy perspectives and cognitive behavioural approaches developed further too, adding ever-more sophisticated, yet contradictory, perspectives to the non-biological approaches to mental distress.[26] Only *innovative conceptual deconstruction* will be looked at here.

The evolving process in the 1980s and 1990s has perhaps been less vocal than the parallel process in the 1960s and 1970s, but in some ways it has been more painstaking and no less important. It has come more from psychologists and some psychiatrists than from sociologists and social workers on the one hand, and directly from users (and much less from relatives) on the other hand. A culmination of the process can be detected towards the end of the 1980s and the early 1990s.

In *Reconstructing Schizophrenia*[27] it is proposed that the concept of schizophrenia as used in psychiatry is flawed philosophically and methodologically to the point that it should be thrown out of everyday use. While the contributors do not necessarily share the same viewpoint as to the definition of schizophrenia and its origins, they share the overall methodological view and point out the following flaws in the concept of Schizophrenia as a diagnostic category:

- The inconsistency of the concept.
- Its initial poor methodological base (for example symptoms exhibited by people labelled as suffering from schizophrenia were elevated to become the signs of schizophrenia in others; symptoms in common with other diagnostic categories such as depression were ignored; symptoms of organic illnesses suffered by these people were attributed to schizophrenia).
- The unidimensional approach to the concept of disease and to a phenomenon such as schizophrenia, which is patently multidimensional (*if* it exists at all).
- The inability to distinguish between symptoms and syndromes, symptoms and causes.
- The disregard of people's life experiences and 'careers' as mental patients.
- The continuing disregard of research findings that do not prove what psychiatrists want to hear.

However, while proposing pointers as to how to research the issue further, to date the critique has not led to the development of an alternative conceptual framework.

A less analytical report, but rich in material, is the largest and longest European follow-up of people diagnosed as suffering from schizophrenia, carried out by Ciompi and his colleagues in Switzerland.[28] They too have come to the conclusion that the concept of schizophrenia lacks validity given the enormous variations in outcomes and life experiences, and that the key to understanding 'it' lies in making sense of people's individual life patterns. Many user groups would endorse such a conclusion. As will be outlined below, Ciompi's latest attempt to come up with an *integrated* concept (affect logic) as an explanation of schizophrenia is not convincing.[29]

'Expressed emotions' was developed from the end of the 1970s and throughout the 1980s by researchers and practitioners interested in the issue of family interaction for people diagnosed as suffering from schizophrenia.[30] The concept is based on the findings that the *style* of communication in families is likely to influence the likelihood of a relapse into schizophrenic crisis, or prevent such a relapse. The researchers on expressed emotions did not doubt the validity of the concept of schizophrenia, nor its assumed biological aetiology.

The existence of a family communication style that is hostile and critical has thus been found but not explained. Once found it was put to use in an educational programme aimed at providing relatives and sufferers with information about schizophrenia as a disease and introducing new coping strategies that focused on reducing friction and hostile critical comments.[31] The use of an educational framework is an extension of cognitive behavioral approaches that were especially utilised in constructing a conceptual framework and intervention strategies concerning depression in the 1970s and early 1980s, around key components such as learned helplessness and hopelessness.[32]

Both the basic research and the educational programme have been tried in a number of European countries (Britain, Germany, Greece, Italy and Spain) and outside Europe, with a high rate of repeated findings (even though dissenting findings have been found.[33] However the importance of expressed emotions to the deconstruction of the psychiatric diagnostic system has not been taken up by its developers, for the obvious reason that they do not doubt the validity of the diagnostic system. The research conducted by them does not shed light on whether or not the disruptive style of communication predated the development of the symptoms, as they were not interested in exploring this issue. In an earlier study by Leff and Hirsch,[34] which was a replication of research conducted by Wynne and Singer in the United States on defects of communication in similar families (as well as a number of other families, with different disabilities), the British group did not find evidence to prove the hypothesis of specific defects in communication typifying families of people with schizophrenia.

The contribution of expressed emotions to the conceptual deconstruction of mental illness seems to me to lie in emphasising the limit of a purely biological approach to schizophrenia, or any other psychiatric diagnostic category for that matter. It would have been useful if expressed emotions had not been treated just as an auxiliary concept and technique, but as a conceptual tool with which to reinvestigate the diagnostic system, a system that usually does not take family interaction into an etiological account.

Affect logic

Ciompi[35] has recently proposed an integrative concept that he calls 'affect logic'. He suggests that schizophrenia develops within an evolutionary model. At the first phase a specific affective–cognitive vulnerability is established, due to interacting genetic and psychosocial influences. Through a process of decompensation, psychosis is developed. Whether or not the psychosis remains depends on a large number of individual and contextual variables. Ciompi does not rule out complete remission, or any intermittent possibility. As Brown and Harris have demonstrated in their study of depression among women,[36] vulnerability comes directly out of a psychosocial context.

While integrative concepts are very rare in the field of mental distress and are therefore extremely attractive, it is difficult to see how this particular concept could advance our understanding beyond acceptance that every factor in life interacts with other factors. In the end Ciompi seems to rely on the notion of 'limbopathy', that is, reduced brain metabolic function is the first differentiating factor between those who are likely to develop schizophrenia and those who will not. Surely such a reductionist explanation – for which there is little evidence – does not enhance the integrative assumption with which he begins.

The main missing links in Ciompi's analysis are the *critical* conditions, events or contexts that generate what is described as 'schizophrenia', beyond the rather rudimentary proposal that repetitive concrete actions lead to the creation of the psyche (described as a complex hierarchy of affective–cognitive systems of reference). If such a link does not exist, perhaps there is no justification in continuing to treat as one category the multitude of behaviours and feelings currently attributed to schizophrenia.

Challenging behaviour

The concept of *challenging behaviour* is currently replacing the conceptual constructs of *inadequate personality* and *psychopathy* in Britain, but not in the rest of Europe, where neither terms is in frequent use.

Challenging behaviour implies behaviour that is socially unacceptable and is perceived to be either aggressive or embarrassing to others. Ciponi[37] defines it as-a behaviour may be a problem if it satisfies some or all of the following criteria:

1. The behaviour itself or its severity is inappropriate given a person's age and level of development.
2. The behaviour is dangerous either to the person him-or herself or to others.
3. The behaviour constitutes a significant additional handicap for the person by interfering with the learning of new skills or by excluding the person from important learning opportunities.
4. The behaviour causes significant stress to the lives of those who live and work with the person and impairs the quality of their lives to an unreasonable degree.
5. The behaviour is contrary to social norms.

Thus the focus shifts from the person to that of his/her behaviour, a shift that on its own reflects a less over-generalising and stigmatising approach. The reliance on social norms as the benchmark for diagnostic decisions continues, as does the judgement that some behaviours are more self-defeating than others.

On the face of it is difficult to understand why such a behaviour is seen as a psychiatric category, unless it is assumed that it reflects an underlying mental distress problem. Even seeing it as a symptom does not justify labelling it as a diagnostic category, as it can – and indeed does – accompany a number of existing diagnostic labels, such as manic behaviour, hysteria and schizophrenia. A related issue is whether or not the person can help behaving in this way, that is whether she/he is responsible for the behaviour and can control it.

The concept was originally developed in the field of learning difficulties, where the issue of whether a person is likely to suffer from both learning difficulties and non-psychotic mental distress had to be confronted in conjunction with the degree of self-responsibility that can be expected from a person with learning difficulties. The concept has since been elaborated by psychologists and psychiatrists with a behavioural perspective,[38] where there is less interest in underlying causes and more interest in defining and changing behaviour. By focusing on definitions and changes to a specific behavioural pattern they might also have hoped to avoid labelling people, aware that labelling took place when either psychopathy or inadequate personality were used.

The following explanatory frameworks have been proposed to account for the origins of challenging behaviour:[39]

- neurological deficits (for example frontal lobe seizure);
- metabolic abnormality;
- a way of communicating for people who find it difficult to be heard otherwise;
- a mental illness.

So far, proof of any of the above in the case of people who do not have learning difficulties or epilepsy is lacking.

The incentive to develop a framework for tackling such behaviours has been the policy of hospital closure, resettlement and prevention, and the reinstitutionalisation of both children and adults with learning difficulties. The same incentive exists for mental health workers and planners, but perhaps in an even more urgent form, given the fears concerning resettlement and limited hospital admissions. This laudable motivation has perhaps led to acceptance of what can at best be described as a lousy conceptual construct in its internal logic, validity and reliability. As with the definition of psychopathy in the British Mental Health Act of 1959, socially unacceptable behaviour that is not criminal is being boxed into a mental illness category to fill the gap created by freeing a residual category of people from another form of social control (the total institution).

Yet the lively public debate that took place between 1957 and 1959 as to whether psychopathy should become a mental illness category is not in evidence in the 1990s, apart from the more limited debate on the ethical issues of the proposed community supervision order and its usefulness.[40] The absence of a debate on the validity of the category is partly related to its location within the context of planning future services for resettled users and future clients, that is, it has become a implementation 'technical' issue. However the readiness of planners to take for granted this new category, which has no proven track record, reflects the overwhelming fear of socially unacceptable behaviour leading to the unquestioned wish to construct settings in which it will be enclosed and hidden from the public gaze.

In the process of catering for this potential threat, important conceptual questions are not being asked, let alone investigated. The doubts expressed in the 1950s on both the validity of the concept and the usefulness of interventions related to it are no less valid in the 1990s, including the possibility of accepting that, unless criminal, such behaviour has to be looked at within the context in which the specific individual exhibiting it lives, rather than in the global labelling form that the new category embraces.

Why is the new category missing from the European scene? Perhaps for the same reason that we have not seen the demonisation of the new long stay in Europe – in part due to an attitudinal change and in part due to the realisation of the serious limitations of the psychiatric diagnostic system, as well as the lower level of focus on law and order issues in other European countries.

Accepting voices

Romme and Escher's edited volume *Accepting Voices*[41] is the culmination of an investigation carried out since 1986, initially in the Netherlands but now including Britain, into the phenomenon of hearing voices. In traditional psychiatry hearing voices is one of the differentiating symptoms for psychosis, especially schizophrenia. Psychiatric texts provide examples of how voices have tormented people and driven them either to self-harm or to harm others.[42]

In the mid-1980s Professor Romme, a psychiatrist from the University of Limburg in the Netherlands, stumbled across a woman service user who was tormented by the voices she was hearing, a condition not alleviated by the medication she took regularly. The only comfort she got was from the knowledge that hearing voices was a normal practice in ancient times. Professor Romme and the client decided to explore the baffling issue of voices with other people hearing them. From one-to-one meetings they began small group meetings, and were later given the opportunity to appear on Dutch television and ask for people who had heard voices to contact them. 700 people responded, and many of them attended a conference that took place some time later.

Romme and Escher (a journalist who also worked at the University of Limburg) were particularly interested to learn from the users attending the conference, and later from those who replied to a detailed questionnaire, that while two thirds were distressed by the voices, another third found them helpful. Further discussion and research revealed more about the nature of the voices and the coping strategies available to those who hear distressing messages.

The new approach to hearing voices suggests that:

- Users are aware that the voices do not represent the presence of a real person, even when they are attributed to a real person.
- Some such voices can be beneficial, perceived as an 'alter ego', the complimentary part of oneself, or as an advice giver.
- People are proud to have the extraordinary ability of hearing voices.
- There are a number of useful coping mechanisms to control the impact of negative messages and thus avoid medication.
- Users can train others to achieve a better understanding and the ability to cope.

The Dutch and British Hearing Voices Networks are loose networks of people who are ready to take hearing voices seriously, offer mutual support, and explore together this vexing and fascinating issue.

It is clear from the evidence produced in the book edited by Romme and Escher that hearing voices is not limited to mental health service users, or to a particular diagnostic category, or to being mentally ill. It is also clear that it is a live phenomenon in the post-modern era in which we live, even though most of us have internalised the message that hearing voices is a clear-cut sign of serious mentally illness. While for some people hearing voices relates to a religious experience, for others it is part of a gift of understanding life in a different way from that available to the majority. That so many people have come forward to declare that they hear voices *without being perceived as mentally ill by themselves or by others, including professionals*, highlights that to confine hearing voices to a psychiatric symptom is only to distort their reality.

Here is how one woman describes some of her experiences in Romme's and Escher's collection:[43]

> Before discussing how hearing voices has affected my life, let me introduce myself. I am a woman of 61, married, with a son and daughter-in-law and two grandchildren. For many years, I successfully combined a career as a social worker with running a home and raising a family until I was physically incapacitated. I now receive state sickness benefit.
> I heard voices since childhood. They foretell the future, as well as advising and directing me. I received my first definite message at the age of nine. We were living in a harbour town at the time, and one day a Greek tanker moored in the harbour began to explode. The noise of the first explosion was so loud that it carried to my school. My father was a member of the fire brigade and rushed to the scene. ... Several hours later, I heard an inner voice say: 'your father will return', and told my mother about this. Just then, our neighbour came in and said that the tanker was expected to blow up completely. I was terribly afraid, but again I clearly heard a voice repeat: 'Your father will return'. This turned out to be the truth: a complete stranger grabbed hold of my father and pulled him clear, while a colleague standing next to him was killed by flying iron bars.
> I kept quiet about this incident, though I heard voices more and more frequently. I was puzzled by their significance – I did not believe in spirits – and did not know whether to resist them. They were there all the time, which I found tiring. Finally, my only hope of relief was to confide in my parents. They did not understand, but did not make fun of me; they listened attentively, although they were unable to advise me what to do.
> I have never ceased to hear voices. They are intrusive, but friendly; they heighten my awareness, and are part and parcel of me. ... The voices have transformed my life, and I ask you to respect that fact.

Mainstream psychiatry has yet to take into account the significance of this new – and old – evidence. Taking it into account would mean accepting that hearing voices *per se* is not a symptom of mental illness, but an extension of our perception. It may be part of a mental illness insofar as voices may reflect conflict and rejection, anger and revenge, or unjustified superiority. At the same time hearing voices may be part of tuning into a more collective, unconscious, stream of awareness.

Writing as someone who has not (so far) heard voices, as someone who is not a believer in any religion, I am aware that accepting the existence of voices as a non-symptomatic phenomenon means that the psychiatric diagnostic system is insufficiently sensitive to minority experiences and too hasty to judge any such experience as a pathology. In doing so mainstream psychiatry is reducing people's experiences to a disease and treating them inappropriately, to their detriment and our general impoverishment. Furthermore it has failed miserably to *learn from users' experiences*, which are continuously invalidated. By doing so, mainstream psychiatry has harmed people where it intended to help them, through the combined impact of labelling and medication. Instead mental health professionals need to learn a lot more from users, as well as from other voice hearers in Western and non-Western societies, about hearing voices, coping with negative voices and putting to good use the positive messages.

Thus accepting voices not only means redressing the imbalance of power relations between professionals and users, but also reexamining the models of understanding reality that are presently prominent in Western psychiatry, for they have been found wanting.

Romme and other contributors also outline a number of coping strategies that can be learned and that enhance the individual's control over his/her environment, without the use of medication (for a description of this approach see Chapter 4).

Sexual abuse as an everyday phenomenon

Writing about sexual abuse in 1994, it seems that we have come a long way from Freud's difficulty in accepting that the illicit sexual relations described by some of his clients actually took place.

Despite Masson's attack on psychoanalysis for this denial, and on psychotherapy in general for being a brainwashing tool,[44] it is relevant to note that:

1. The attempt to conceptually understand sexual abuse in its mental health and distress concept has been largely undertaken by psychoanalytically inclined professionals.
2. The psychotherapists who work with victims of sexual abuse and with perpetrators of such abuse to find ways of leading

a more positive life, and of coming to terms with what has happened and its terrible impact, are mostly (but by no means exclusively) of psychoanalytic orientation.

This can perhaps be explained by the guilt felt by psychoanalysts at Freud's mistake, but even more by the fact that psychoanalysis remains rooted in the junction between rationality and irrationality, sexuality and conformity to social norms, internal and external logic and interaction, conscious and unconscious experiences.

Reliable figures on the frequency of abuse are impossible to come by. Likewise in many cases it is not possible to validate whether or not children and adults are speaking the truth, or the full truth. Nevertheless the persistence of exposure of abuse across different social classes and Western countries makes it equally impossible to continue to deny that it does happen in our midst, and perhaps more often than we would like to believe.

Accepting that sexual abuse does take place leaves all of us with a collective guilt that is difficult to bear, for we have all been socialised to accept incest as taboo, that children do not have forced sexual relations, and that people have a right to sexual relations without violence. Our ingrained belief that none of these take place is being put into question by the presence of sexual abuse in everyday life.

No less fundamentally, the existence of sexual abuse puts into also question the meaning of *love*, especially *unconditional* love between parents and children. It also raises once more the unresolved issue of the relationship between love and sexuality, and between sexuality and social norms.

One of the least surprising revelations is the existence of sexual abuse in total institutions for people with learning difficulties and mental illness, for brutality in such places could have been predicted in advance.[45] Yet it is an aspect that professionals do not wish to discuss, as it implies a clear breach of professional ethics and trust.

The existence of ritualised sexual abuse – called satanic abuse by some – is even more incredible and difficult to believe and accept. In Britain it has recently been the subject of a government sponsored inquiry by a highly reputed anthropologist, who concluded that *organised* abuse exists, but not necessarily *ritualised* abuse. To an outsider to the field of sexual abuse like myself, this distinction seems not that important when compared with the horrors of systematic physical, sexual and emotional abuse by more than one person, described in rather graphic terms by a number of people whose stories have been corroborated.[46]

Thus an intricate combination of conceptual and ethical issues, as yet far from fully understood and explained, has come to the fore in this case (as elsewhere in mental health, yet somehow even stronger). The conceptual response has been innovative in terms of the attempt to put together the different pieces of the puzzle, by mapping the process of sorting out the ethical dilemmas that sexual abuse raises from the perspective of the victim on the one hand, and the perpetrator on the other.[47] *Victims* seem to go through an initial process that includes shock, fear, fascination, a sense of being selected that carries with it a measure of power as well as of being punished for sins committed earlier, of being invaded, brutalised, and dirty for ever.

The high level of ambiguity we find among other types of victim (for example, of torture, of rape by an unknown outsider) is also found here. This includes experiencing guilt, shame, complicity and unworthiness, and identifying with the aggressor. Often victims are self-mutilating, enter highly destructive relationships, lack self-confidence and/or withdraw into mental illness and at times into learning difficulties.

In understanding *perpetrators* too we have to be able to enter their conceptual and belief systems without abandoning our own systems, however remote and loathed their framework may seem to us. Perpetrators tend to convince themselves gradually that there is nothing wrong with what they are doing; that the child/weaker adult is not that hurt; that the victim is in fact enjoying the relationship; that the relationship is 'special'; that the attraction is mutual; that they – and only they – truly love the child/adult.

Perpetrators are understood as adults who have often been damaged as children themselves, and therefore have not in fact internalised the most fundamental social norms in the way the rest of us have; who are unable to distinguish between their desire and the pain of others; who derive pleasure from infringing social norms and from causing pain; who often feel impotent socially and sexually in their relations with adults; who are fascinated by infringing social norms and letting themselves be ruled by desire only; who find that the secrecy attached enhances their pleasure. Most perpetrators are not recognised as mentally ill, and no one diagnostic category fits this type of abnormal behaviour.

The third category – that is they *partners* or relatives of abusive perpetrators, especially parents – have been looked at less, and often in a stereotypical and dismissive way. While some have been accused of complicity by those abused, the majority have been described as passive, weak partners who are verbally and physically intimidated by the abuser. Others have been depicted as equally attracted to the unspeakable.

The difficulties inherent in an attempt to understand unimaginable situations and the process workers have to go through to be able to listen, believe, accept and tolerate pain and self-loathing as an inevitable part of the purifying process, or complete denial, will be looked at in Chapter 6, as will the quality of the emotional impact that such a task has on us as workers and human beings.

A fourth, and often unspoken of category consists of workers in the caring professions who abuse their clients, often in a residential setting. In such a setting the dependency of the client on the worker looms large. The abuse here is not only of the person for whose welfare the worker is responsible, but also of professional ethics and the social mandate given to the worker. Apart from expressions of horror, no systematic attempt has been made to understand such transgressions, and we often comfort ourselves with the fact that most of the workers found guilty of abuse have been unqualified professionals.

The conceptual implications of the emergence of users and relatives as stakeholders

The transformation of users and relatives into stakeholders, and the processes leading to it, are described in Chapter 4. In this section the focus is on the conceptual implications of this development.

The emergence of mental health service users as partners to the rethinking of these services and the implementation of the rethinking is closely related to a number of factors, such as:

- their greater social visibility in the wake of hospital closure;
- the impact of the demarginalisation process in Italy, in-

fluenced by the new social movements that emerged in the 1960s, and the rekindled interest in citizen participation in Britain;
- the impact of the social role valorisation approach and the US user movement;
- the focus on consumers by the British and Dutch governments;
- the relative success of the Dutch user organisations in having a formally accepted presence within the Dutch hospital system as well as social policy planning structures.[48]

It is relevant and interesting to note that most of the spokespersons and activists in the user movement are people who are categorised as continued care clients, not those suffering from mild distress or a one-off episode of mental breakdown. This highlights the fact that the assumed potential of continued care clients is not a myth. Is involvement in the user movement a way of consolidating a threatened identity, through building a positive group identity? It is clearly a choice that relatively few people take up, while the majority prefer to use the *passing* coping strategy, that is, to hide the existence of mental distress.

As Viv Lindow has suggested,[49] the British user movement has been *reactive* (for example to proposals concerning community supervision orders), *proactive* (for example in proposing refuge facilities in the community as alternatives to hospitalisation, in its contribution to training social workers and nurses), and *creative* (for example the very creation of the user movement; the rethinking and mutual support around hearing voices, described above). Conceptually the users' views highlight the fact that the subjective and intersubjective experiences of both mental illness and the psychiatric system are as important and as valid as professional perspectives, but they are often *different*, and are much less complementary than those of professionals when evaluating the latter's contribution. Furthermore, their conceptual contribution has forced us to look at issues of interpersonal relationships, social positions and attitudes as underlying most crisis reactions and blocking reintegration.

Their descriptions of institutional life have enabled us to fathom the sense of isolation and exclusion that prevail in these places. The actual and potential damage of overuse of medication has also been highlighted by some user groups, as have the possible alternatives to medication.

The work carried out on understanding eating problems and self-harm[50] has illustrated the interaction between inner states and physical appearance; controlling one's weight or self-harm as a desperate attempt to feel in control over something important to one's own identity, coupled with the wish for purification. Within this approach people should retain the right to starve to death or to mutilate and eventually kill themselves, a rather unpalatable belief for most of us.

However, on the whole the user movement has perhaps paid insufficient attention to issues relating to individual responsibility, risk, violence, relatives and body–mind interaction.

Relatives

So far little conceptual development has taken place in terms of understanding the complexity of relatives' experiences of their Kinsperson's mental distress, of mental illness itself, and of being at the receiving end of the professional system. This paucity of progress relates in part to the greater focus on direct users, and to the way relatives prefer to portray themselves in straightforward terms that are often very clear-cut and unambiguous.[51]

In actively campaigning for a halt to hospital closure rather than the development of an alternative framework, relatives' groups have often allied themselves with traditional psychiatry and alienated themselves from user groups. The wish of relatives to look for simple explanations and solutions is understandable, as is the preference for biological explanations that stress the lack of a role for family interaction in the context of mental distress. Yet it has led to a very reductionist approach to mental illness, to the people suffering from it, to potential solutions, and consequently to the relatives themselves.

The research on family burden[52] illustrates this oversimplified approach in isolating an important single issue out of an interactive and complex context. The issues of how to make sense of the major mental breakdown of someone close to you, of their failure to return to the level of functioning you were used to (which feels as if it is going to last forever), of their expression of hostility towards but dependency on you, and of professionals giving you the feeling that you are responsible for what has happened/will happen, are still to be properly researched. A promising beginning has recently been made through an oral history approach in which relatives have been asked to talk about their experiences, often more than once.[53] This study illustrates the depth of the emotional ties that relatives have even with users with whom they do not live, their sense of obligation, and the mixture of meanings they give to the mental illness, often holding contradictory views simultaneously.

It might prove productive to apply the concept of threatened identities (discussed earlier in this chapter) not only to service users but to relatives too. Relatives' social and personal identities are threatened by the close proximidy of mental illness, as this raises the issue of whether they will be the next to succumb to this fate, of whether the stigma attached to mental illness will rub off on them, of whether they are internalising the stigma (for example by reducing social contact, by not inviting people to their home in order to avoid embarrassment, by avoiding disclosure of the fact that a family member is mentally ill) and responding to it by adopting one of the coping strategies outlined in Table 2.1 above. As with users, the decision to become a member of a relatives' group, or an activist in the relatives' movement, requires a decision that being a relative of a person suffering from mental illness *is* part of one's identity.

Alison Wertheim's book *A Special Scar* tells the stories of relatives of people who have committed suicide, the final act of despair and defiance that leaves relatives to pick up the pieces. The book illustrates the process of shame, guilt and self-exploration, as well as continuing to live after such a shattering experience. The text shows that there are no simple or uniform resolutions, only painful individualised ways of coming to terms with what has happened, at times including relief that it has all come to an end

Missing conceptual development

An integrative approach

Virtually no conceptual work has been carried out on creating an integrative approach to mental distress, or on genuine user and carer participation in the conceptual perspectives of professional knowledge. This is illustrated in particular by the lack of focus on mental health in terms of what it means beyond the absence of illness, of the factors that lead to it, sustain it or stop it from materialising.

In the 1970s Garmezy proposed that some children of parents suffering from schizophrenia demonstrate *resilience* factors.[54] Antonovsky[55] has proposed that *salutogenic* factors exist in relation to health in general, which are focused on retaining an overall integrative perspective of life, even in the face of adversity. We have all come across such people; we are also aware that under extreme conditions of deprivation and humiliation most people do not develop psychiatric symptoms, and some of them are able to support others at considerable risk to themselves. Still others suggest that the spiritual aspect of our lives is the core of mental health. Yet conceptual work on mental health is still to be undertaken.

The related place of *ethics* as guiding the development of conceptual knowledge has remained unclear and blurred, with the exceptions of the SRV approach and that of action research.[56]

The concept of innovation

Despite the considerable degree of innovation in mental health systems that has taken place since the early 1980s in Western Europe, little has been developed in terms of creating a conceptual framework for understanding *innovation*. Such a framework would include a better understanding of the specific issues that require innovation, the specific issues faced by innovators in mental health services and the issues they share with innovators in related fields.

So far, most of the conceptual framework has been borrowed from organisational management approaches to public and private sector enterprises.[57] For this to be effective, mental health innovators need to know what they are looking for. Some of the lessons of *action research* are directly applicable to mental health innovation. This is particularly the case when the participation of the major stakeholders is to be encouraged, as action research is based on activating participants, of involving participants in identifying issues to be acted upon and desirable solutions, as well as contributing to the process of action and evaluation.

In action research both action and evaluation are moved from being imposed from above (employers, the state) or from afar (by researchers). In changing the traditional relationships between the participants, in innovation new freedoms and new constraints are encountered, as power relationships and the very definition of what is *valuable knowledge* change. The research on voices described above in the section on the conceptual deconstruction of mental illness provides an apt example of such changes. Zeelen, van der Meer and van de Graaf [58] have also highlighted how being available as researchers to patients and staff in an action research project in a psychiatric hospital in Holland enables hitherto hidden perspectives to come to light, including the role of service users and ex-users as researchers.

Changes in power and professionalism

Most of the changes in the mental health services that have taken place since 1980 have led to changes in the power relationships among the different stakeholders and within groups of stakeholders (for example the relative power given to nurses versus the power taken away from psychiatrists, described in Chapter 6, and the pressure power taken by relatives and users, described in Chapter 4).

These changes – including those in power relations – have also led to some changes in views about professionalism, about how professionals should be trained and what they should be providing, including the increasing role of non-professionally qualified workers (see Chapters 1 and 6). However, while recognised, these changes have been only partially analysed and investigated.[59] The inherent conservative and defensive position of those afraid of losing power or of change may be one of the reasons for the paucity of research in this area. The existing research is looked at in Chapter 6, as most of it relates to professionals.

The journey through the most innovative conceptual developments in the 1980–95 period, outlined above, has revealed some promising avenues for further work, rather than described completed developments. It has also highlighted the fact that the validity of some of our cherished systems of knowledge should be seriously questioned and some elements discard. Gaps in our existing knowledge have been identified, as well as the considerable degree of discomfort that some of the new concepts bring with them.

3
Ethnicity and Gender as Issues for Stakeholders in Mental Distress Services

Introduction: ethnicity and gender as central identity markers

Ethnicity is defined as cultural characteristics that are perceived as differentiating one social group from another.[1] Membership of an ethnic group is a central component of defining individual and group identity, as it incorporates personal and collective history, culture, language and religion, apart from acting as a marker of differences. As such it applies to each and every person, to ethnic minorities and majorities, across the colour divide. All European societies consist of more than one ethnic group, and therefore the issue of majority and minority ethnic group relationships and identities arises for all of them.

Mixed race people, or people of mixed ethnic background, are a subgroup that is presented with additional issues of identity, namely being able, in principle at least, to choose their ethnic identity and/or to live with an ongoing conflict, with two identities, or to create their own mixture. In reality they are confronted with a number of impositions and pressures to conform to choices made by others on their behalf. They may also have to pay the price of not being accepted by one or both ethnic groups.

Gender is the construction of the social and personal connotations of the differences between the sexes.[2] Gender too is a central component of our personal and group identity, and of our social relations. Due to its base within undisputed biological differences it may be seen as even more crucial than ethnicity at the psychological level. However, as the centrality of a component may change according to the specific context, this is not necessarily the case at times.

Often both ethnicity and gender are used as power markers and brokers. Ethnicity and gender interact at more than one level, such as in differentiating further the issues that women and men from a specific ethnic group may face, versus the shared issues. Likewise gender may unite people across ethnic differences, as has been the case in the women's movement. Both ethnicity and gender are influenced by a number of additional factors, some of which are shared (such as class, the family, the state) and some of which are specific to either ethnicity or gender.

Racism and sexuality are subdimensions of ethnicity and gender.[3] Both racism and sexuality are important elements in the interaction between ethnicity and gender on the one hand, and the interaction of the two latter components in the context of mental health and illness on the other. Both racism and sexuality influence our personal perceptions, feelings and actions, and act as determinants of the opportunities and constraints confronted by us within the society in which we live.

Zlata was admitted to a unit for adolescents after a self-harm attempt in January 1993. She is a good looking, 21 year old woman who lives with her mother and younger brother in a refugee camp in Ljublijana, the capital of Slovenia. They have not heard from the father or the older brother since they left them behind in Bosnia five months previously. In Bosnia she had worked in an office as a junior clerk. She had had a boyfriend

Table 3.1 Matrix of ethnicity and gender in the context of mental distress

The elements and dimensions, and the inter-relationships between them, which should be taken into account here includes:

ELEMENTS	DIMENSIONS		E R M G S R F S LP P I G S
*ethnicity;			
*racism;		MH	
*migration;			
*gender;		MD	
*sexuality;	mental health		
*reproduction	vs.	MI	
*the family;	mental distress		
*the state;	mental illness	MHS	
*lay people;	mental health services		
*professionals;			
*individuals;			
*groups;			
*societies.			

and an active social life. The camp is situated in the grounds of an old army barracks. Refugees are not allowed to work and have to be within the confines of the camp from the early evening.

No psychiatric diagnosis has been made of Zlata, or symptoms identified. The doctor was ready to discharge her when she began to cry and explained how boring life was in the camp, how it was much more interesting in the unit. Not knowing what to do, the doctor allowed her to stay for a few more days. He promised her that she would be invited to the forthcoming party at the unit. When I suggested that it might benefit both sides if she were to befriend some of the unit's long-term residents, I could see the look of disbelief in the eyes of the people around me.

Given her current life circumstances, Zlata is likely to become more mentally distressed if she continues to stay in the camp; unless the regime there changes dramatically to provide her with a more meaningful life and allows her to work through her recent traumatic experiences. 'Ethnic cleansing' policies forced her to leave her birthplace, but because she is Bosnian she feels (and *is* to an extent) unwelcomed in Slovenia too, even though the two countries were part of Yugoslavia until three years ago. Being a woman it was assumed that she should leave rather than stay as her older brother did. Her mother disapproves of her attempts to chat up the few young Slovenian men that she has met since arriving; the days have no structure; she has no money whatsoever; she has no new clothes, only handouts. . . . Zluta's current experience encapuslates the combined impact of ethnicity and gender within the context of a nationalistic conflict, in which both characteristics become handicaps.

There is sufficient evidence to demonstrate that members of ethnic minorities are more likely than the majority to:[4]

1. be diagnosed as suffering from psychosis;
2. be admitted to hospital, and on a compulsory order;
3. remain for longer periods in hospital;
4. be treated with medication, rather than by counselling or social rehabilitation.

However these probabilities are not evenly distributed among different ethnic minorities. In France, North Africans have a higher rate of identified mental distress than Africans. In Britain, Irish and Afro-Caribbean people top the list, not only in having higher rates than other groups, but also in having rates that are much higher than could have been predicted by their percentage in the population. People from the Indian subcontinent are at the bottom of this list.[5] Furthermore the rate of psychosis and hospital admissions among white, Christian, British people is higher than the rate of the Asian population.

The fact that Irish people top the list highlights the importance of ethnicity *vis-à-vis* racism. Yet it would be misleading to assume that the only reason for the high rate of mental illness and hospital admission of this group pertains to ethnicity. It definitely pertains to the specific history of the Anglo–Irish relationship, which is marred not only by colonialism and oppression, but also by the concentration of Irish people in Britain among the working class. The fact that the parallel rates in Ireland are also high in comparison with other European countries[6] has to be taken into account too. This finding has been explained by some as due to genetic predisposition, and by others as the result of a turbulent history.

A different picture emerges when looking at the Afro-Caribbean group. At home this group has a much lower rate of both psychosis and hospital admission than in Britain. Racism and frustration at unfulfilled expectations are clearly at play. In addition schizophrenia is diagnosed more frequently among young Afro-Caribbean men, and this is likely to be related to lay beliefs about their sexual prowess and their tendency to act violently.

Police involvement in compulsory admission is much more noticeable in relation to this group than to other ethnic subgroups, raising the possibility that the police are both called in by lay people and reflect lay people's views. At the same time there is no evidence to suggest that the lead given by the police is not followed by the professionals involved, namely psychiatrists and social workers.[7]

The lower rate of Asian people is explained in part by the middle-class origin of some of them, their reluctance to use Eurocentric services, and the use of alternative healers within their communities.

A number of psychiatrists have proposed that genetic predisposition lies at the core of this situation. A rate of schizophrenia among second generation Afro-Caribbeans (in and out of hospital) that was 12 times higher than that of the general population was found in a Nottingham study conducted by Harrison et al. in the 1980s.[8] Similarly, a study carried out in Manchester by Thomas et al.[9] in 1991 found that Afro-Caribbeans born in Britain have a much higher rate than British-and European-born people, unlike members of Asian groups. Thomas et al. noted that the rate of unemployment was much higher among British-born Afro-Caribbeans than among the two other groups, and that Afro-Caribbean parents had a lower rate of schizophrenia. Nevertheless he too proposed a genetic explanation.

Those who do not espouse the genetic explanation have proposed that the high diagnosis of schizophrenia among Afro-Caribbean men is due to one of the following:[10]

- Misdiagnosis
- Racism
- Reflection of true incidence

Migration and mental distress

As suggested above, ethnic minorities begin to emerge after members of these groups have migrated to a 'host' country. The experience of migration by choice is one of disruption, but also of hope and an expectation of doing better than was possible in the country of origin. While the majority in the new country usually expect the newcomers to adapt to the majority's way of living, the immigrants are confronted with the dilemma of living within and between two cultures, and of the need to take decisions as to whether they want to become 'acculturated' to the majority's culture and/or retain their original culture, or opt for a mixture of both cultures.

While up to the 1970s it was assumed that immigrants would have a higher rate of mental illness than natives because of the crisis of immigration, more recent statistics do not corroborate these assumptions when variables such as class and educational level are included.[11]

The push for the assimilation of immigrants continues to exist throughout Europe, despite formal acceptance of the desirability of pluralistic coexistence. This is particularly true of immigrants' children born in the adopted country. This issue applies to both white and black ethnic minorities, and will be illustrated here in its mental distress context through the Greek community in Britain.

There are about 160 000 Greek people in Britain, most of whom came from Cyprus (which was ruled by Britain until the early 1970s). It is an ethnic group that is known for retaining its cohesiveness and cultural values, and for its members' tendency to live in close geographic proximity, not only those in Britain but also those in the Netherlands and the United States.[12] This should have led to a high degree of conflict with the British native majority, and consequently to a higher incidence of mental illness. On the other hand strength and mutual support can be gained by continuing to adhere to particular cultural values that are shared by a group of people. The economic success of a substantial number of members of this community and the lack of racism towards it (even though prejudices abound) are additional important variables on the plus side.

On the whole the Greek community does have a lower rate of mental illness than British natives, and most other European and non-European groupings in Britain. There is also some evidence to suggest that their rate of identified mental illness is lower than that of Greek people in Cyprus and Athens.[13] At the same time the younger generation in particular is experiencing difficulties in continuing to live within and between two cultures. Some of them are expressing these difficulties through relatively mild psychiatric symptomatology and some somatic symptomatology and by rebelling at school or at home, or in both settings. The bewilderment and frustration experienced by their parents is not – and should not be – classified as mental illness, but definitely merits categorisation as non-clinical mental distress, including depressed, confused and aggressive behaviour.

There are a number of Greek professionals in the British mental health services, including a psychotherapist working in Nafsiyat, a not-for-profit agency specialising in providing psychotherapy to ethnic minorities by members of their own ethnic group. These service provides suggest that while there is a need to understand the culture from which the Greeks in Britain are coming, it is in a way even more important to take into account the family dynamics exhibited in the families of these young people (including the impact of immigration), and the youngsters' personalities, than to assume that the specificity of being Greek is the most important variable to be considered.

The perspective of ethnic minority service users

No systematic research has been undertaken on this aspect, perhaps because it is not perceived as a worthwhile recipient of funding. Therefore the nature of the evidence is anecdotal and idiosyncratic. Existing reports (in writing, on tapes and video) highlight the sense of estrangement between the client from an ethnic minority and the clinician, the sense that the latter is neither interested nor able to understand the subjective experience of the client.[14] Furthermore, recognition that the professional would in any case be unable to sort out the structural elements involved (such as racism and unemployment) is a further barrier to the encounter being helpful. The client comes with his/her experience of being discriminated against in other formal settings, and is not anticipating any other reaction. The presence of mental health workers from one's ethnic community is usually experienced as helpful, but more often than not these workers occupy lower power positions than their white colleagues.

Services provided by their own ethnic group (for example Jewish, Irish, Chinese) are experienced by most clients with relief and lead to a greater (albeit qualified) readiness to trust the service providers. However some people do not identify with their ethnic group or have internalised the view that professionals from the same ethnic background cannot be as good as white professionals.

There are a number of black psychiatrists (usually of Indian origin in Britain; African or North African origin in France; Iranian or Turkish in Germany) and a high proportion of Jewish psychiatrists in most European countries. This demographic distribution reflects the marginalisation of psychiatry within medicine, which makes it easier for foreigners to enter it and attracts those who feel themselves to be marginalised. Only a few of these highly qualified (and middle class) professionals have acknowledged the criticism outlined above and proposed alternative approaches. This state of affairs is hardly surprising, as the socialising impact of being trained to become a doctor or a psychiatrist leads to the internalisation of the medical model, including the distanced relationship between doctor and patient.

A Channel 4 programme made in 1993 focused on Elliott, a 26 year old British-born Afro-Caribbean man. For the last three years he had been in a special hospital. He looked disoriented, fat, 'zomby'-like. Photographs from his secondary school revealed a lively, good looking boy who was winning chess competitions. It appears he suffered from depression at the age of 16, unhelped by – or related to – a teacher who said in front of everyone that Elliott would never make it to the A-levels. He left school at the end of the year, and stayed at home after attempts to get a job led nowhere. He saw a psychologist, and then a psychiatrist. One day his mother left him in charge of his younger sister, whom he tried to help with her homework. They had an argument, and he slapped her. She cried, and the neighbours called the police. The police referred him to a psychiatric hospital. He objected to the admission, and was therefore put in a locked ward.

His next four years were spent in two psychiatric hospitals and a secure unit. He was given phenomenal quantities and combinations of medication, which exceeded the BMA's (British Medical Association) recommended dosage, according to a number of reputable consultant psychiatrists. The prescribing psychiatrist was not reprimanded, but resigned his post and is now working in private practice. All that is left to his parents, apart from weekly visits to a remote place, is to sue the authorities and hope for financial compensation.

This is an *atypical* case in the sense that such a travesty of the Hippocratic oath and such tragic outcomes do not usually happen. But it is a typical example of how black young men are not heard, and how they – and their parents – are overlooked.

Alternatives to traditional Eurocentric perspectives

Conceptual alternatives

Non-Eurocentric approaches to mental health and distress are embedded in spiritual and religious systems that differ considerably from either Greek philosophy or the Judeo–Christian tradition upon which the Eurocentric approach is loosely based.

Most of them are based on the desire for harmony between individual, nature and society. In such harmony the individual is usually a receiving entity and not an initiating actor. While there are important differences between Hinduism, Buddhism,

Confucianism and Islam, the call for acceptance of life as it is, including suffering, personal unhappiness and social injustice, is prevalent in all of them. Mental health is acquired through acceptance of what life has given to one, and mental distress can be the outcome of sin on the part of the individual or someone in his/her family, or of a curse put on him/her by others. Dwelling on one's unhappiness is viewed as signifying a lack of internatlisation of social norms and/or of working towards a higher spiritual level of being, in which desire becomes insignificant.

It would seem that psychological and sociological approaches to mental health and illness are omitted from non-Western approaches no less than they are omitted from traditional psychiatry, at least at the conceptual level.

A very different approach is proposed by thinkers from ethnic minorities who formulated their framework as a result of their encounter with Western thought and Eurocentric psychiatry. Fanon,[15] an Algerian psychiatrist educated within the French system and active in the Algerian struggle against French colonialism, perhaps personifies this development. According to him, life within a colonial system influences the personalities of those colonised, and not only their life circumstances. While individual responses, vary the hallmark of this experience lies in being treated as an intellectually and morally inferior human being in one's own country, and in *internalising* one's sense of inferiority and ambiguity as well as the anger one feels towards oneself and the colonising other. A permanent psychological shadow – or a disability – remains, which may lead to brutalisation of the victim as much as to that of the initial aggressor (the colonising power).

While Fanon did not consider the experience of ethnic minorities from a colonised background living in a European country, others have extended his analysis to such a situation. Holland, Francis and Shashidran[16] have proposed that black ethnic minorities in Britain suffer from a racism that is derived from the colonial experience, and have internalised the very racist stereotypes thrown at them. They argue that mental distress is the outcome of being discriminated against in terms of lack of equal opportunities, as well as the impact of the emotional luggage of living with racism and cultural colonialism.

Alternative interventions

Asian and African intervention methods include the following, side by side with the use of traditional psychiatry and different psychotherapeutic approaches:

1. Community healers, who have usually been trained in the country of origin. Healers are likely to offer a variety of interventions, such as empathy, purification, retreat and meditation, herbal medicines, conflict resolution and placation of the gods.
2. Buddhist establishments offer a non-judgemental environment with elements of retreat and meditation, and people who are ready to listen to the sufferer, as well as to live with him/her and provide everyday support.
3. A focus on the spiritual development of the sufferer.

Those who have taken Fanon's approach on board are likely to offer a mixture of interventions aimed at empowering the sufferer while working with him/her on the underlying psychological and social problems that she he is facing. This is likely to include individual and group psychotherapy, in which issues of racism and colonialism will be discussed in terms of their impact on the person/group and how the person/group can counteract this impact,[17] as well as attempting to provide access to work and training opportunities.

While some of this has been provided within the statutory sector, most of it has been attempted by the not-for-profit sector, by providers from the same ethnic group, often at the initiative of the ethnic community. In offering this range, a combination of methods that were initially developed within a Eurocentric perspective (such as psychotherapy) are taken up in a readopted format and content. Although never stated, the developers of this approach do not seem to be operating from the perspective of accepting nature and society as it is, but from the very Eurocentric position of combatting and changing an unequal society, in part through the empowerment of individuals and groups from ethnic minorities and rejection of the inferior image and position allocated to them by the majority.

In London alone, examples of such services include:

- The Afro-Caribbean mental health association, which pro-

vides counselling, legal representation, housing and befriending schemes (a not-for-profit organisation).
- The Fanon Project, which provides a day centre for Afro-Caribbean people (a not-for-profit organisation).
- The Lambo centre, which offers a day centre to African and Afro-Caribbean users of mental health services and their carers (a statutory service).
- The domestic violence project (Southall Black Sisters, a not-for-profit organisation).
- Nafsiyat: psychotherapy for black people by black professionals (a not-for-profit organisation).
- The Sanctuary: a new service aimed at providing a place of refuge, currently offering art therapy based on Afro-Caribbean tradition, for Afro-Caribbean people by black providers (a statutory service, sponsored jointly by the Departments of Health and Social Services in Lambeth).
- Shanti: a not-for-profit counselling service for black women by black counsellors.
- White City Women in Mental Health Project, where individual psychotherapy and groupwork have been on offer to all women, including black women and white women with black partners, since 1984 (part of a statutory service).

All these initiatives highlight the fact that the need for a change in the input provided to ethnic minorities by the usual services has been recognised by a number of organisations and people, including members of ethnic minorities. Furthermore the direction of the projects outlined above follows more closely the empowerment and reparation approach than merely the provision of more equal services.

At times the approach of these services brings them into conflict with their own ethnic group instead of the white majority. For example the Southall Black Sisters clashed with Asian community leaders on the issue of how to handle domestic violence towards Asian women by Asian men. Not surprisingly the leaders preferred to work behind the scenes and not to denounce attackers or encourage the woman to leave them. Most ethnic minorities members are, understandably, very sensitive about the reputation of their group in the eyes of the external world. Any blemish on the community tends to be ignored or denied as much as possible.

Jewish Care (the Federation of Jewish Welfare Services) provides a range of mental health services to members of the Jewish community, including counselling, psychotherapy, housing, day care, and work on specific themes such as the Holocaust. However their direction is limited to providing a service to an ethnic minority by people who identify with it, rather than making sense of and countering the negative discrimination experiences of the group.

Therefore, although provided by a 'separatist' agency, Jewish Care's practice falls within the brief of the ethnically sensitive approach. Within this approach the focus is not so much on the similarity in the background of the user and the provider as it is on the expectation that the provider will make it his/her business to understand the ethnic background from which the user is coming, as well as the typical experiences of discrimination and inequality, and will incorporate this understanding into the content and format of the service. This approach stems from the assumption that service providers can understand in-depth experiences that they have not gone through personally, due to the commonality in human experiences and in particular to being trained to listen and take on board painful experiences. The tools required for understanding the experience of being a member of an ethnic minority do not differ in principle from those required to understand what it is like to be in a psychotic state, to harm oneself or to be sexually abused – states of being that most professionals (and ordinary people) have not experienced personally.

Gender in Europe

Gender in its application to European women has received considerable attention since the 1960s. Women's groups, national movements, conceptual analysis and research have focused on issues perceived to be at the core of either women's unequal position or on what is unique to women. Legislation in most European countries provides women with equal rights. However, as with ethnic minorities, application of the law does not always follow, especially at the informal level.

In terms of social power, women have made considerable gains and are to be found in power positions in politics, business, administration, the arts, academia and the professions. However, numerically the share of women in the more powerful posts is much lower than their percentage in the population: after all, *women are not a minority*, but constitute roughly half of the populations of all European countries.

Throughout Europe women work outside as well as inside their homes. The statistics demonstrate a range of involvement in full- time work, from 49 per cent for Swedish women to 90 per cent in the case of Italian women.[18] The distribution of full-time and part-time jobs among the different European countries makes for interesting reading on the relationships between economic necessity, job opportunities, availability of child care facilities, cultural preferences and women's choices.

Being a woman in Europe today implies living in a world where women have become much more equal to men than they were in, say, 1945, with greater personal and social expectations as to what constitutes the successful juggling of being the equal of men while remaining different from them. This is particularly the case in relation to juggling family and work lives, caring and achieving, sexuality and motherhood.[19] To a large extent, women continue to be judged by whether they do things as well as men, rather than whether they do them as well as they can/want, or whether men are doing as well as women. As our personal identities reflect to a considerable degree our social identities, most women are likely to have internalised these expectations as their own.

The public emergence of women who are lesbian and men who are homosexual has highlighted the centrality of sexual orientation as a core component within personal and social identities.[20] If anything, this has made the relationship between *sexual orientation* and *gender identity* even more complicated.

Much less has been analysed about men in Western societies, and even less about men in Oriental and post-communist societies.

Gender and mental distress

In most European countries more women than men are identified as suffering from mental distress: more are referred to mental health services or hospitalised, and a much higher number are diagnosed as suffering from illnesses such as depression and senile dementia.[21] On the other hand more men than women enter hospital through compulsory admission and remain for longer periods, and more are diagnosed as suffering from schizophrenia and drug and alcohol abuse.

More married women and single men are to be found among those suffering from mental distress and illness, than single women or married men. The percentage of women admitted to hospital is much higher than the percentage of men after the age of 50, and for men below the age of 35, even though on the whole the women's rate is consistently higher throughout the age range. This finding is related to the impact of life-cycle specific roles, stresses and stereotypes faced by older women on the one hand and by younger men on the other hand.[22] Slovenia is the exception in having the same rate of hospital admission for both men and women.[23]

It is interesting to note in the explainations of these figures that *misdiagnosis* has not been claimed. Unlike ethnic minorities, it is not assumed that male psychiatrists (the majority in the profession) and female psychiatrists (who are trained to diagnose in the same way as their male colleagues) are mistakenly interpreting distress as having made a qualitative jump from unhappiness to psychiatric disturbance. Instead it is assumed that both of those professional subgroups understand women sufficiently and share social definitions of mental health and distress, as well as of how women should behave, think and feel. It is proposed that women's lot in European/Western countries is causing excessive mental distress for women.[24]

Such an explanation is based on the argument that women are faced with too many demands and too many contradictory demands, while at the same time being treated as unequal partners in terms of social power and unreliable partners in terms of emotional balance. Successfully fulfilling the roles of worker, housewife, lover, companion, mother, daughter and friend – beside being oneself – is not only asking a lot, but also expecting different things simultaneously.

It is additionally argued that women are insufficiently supported by men, other women, family members, work colleagues, health professionals, education and social services, and the state. Some would put it in even stronger terms and suggest that women are not only insufficiently supported, but are in fact sabotaged by others in their attempt to meet the impossible demands imposed on them.

Behind the claim of sabotage lies the argument already mentioned above in the discussion on what constitutes mental health, that women's ways of understanding the world and operating in it differ significantly from those of men, and that therefore – given the dominant position of men in our society – this difference (or uniqueness) is repressed and seen as mentally unhealthy.

That women psychiatrists, social workers, nurses and psychologists would collude in such an undertaking is less surprising than it may seem, given the level of socialisation and internalisation that all helping professions, especially medicine, are going through, and the reinforcement due to the congruency between this socialisation and lay views in this specific case.[25] If this is so, then we are looking at misdiagnosis not at the level of individual practitioners, but at the level of the *classifying system* itself and its construction. Although Sheppard has demonstrated that GPs (most of whom are men) refer more women than men for compulsory admission, Davis *et al.* have illustrated that social workers, most of whom are women, do not differ in their approach.[26]

It would therefore seem that, with a few exceptions, the gender of the professional involved does not in itself guarantee a more in-depth understanding and empathy towards users from the same sex any more than professionals from ethnic minorities provide it to users from ethnic minorities.

An alternative explanation for the higher rate of women using mental health services is that this is an artifact of the measurement, rooted in insufficient refinement and the overinclusive nature of epidemiological categories. For example the observation that there is a greater incidence of mental distress among married women does not tell us much about the contribution of marriage to mental distress, as additional factors – such as having children or not, or the degree of satisfaction gained from marital relations – may have a crucial bearing.[27]

Another example relates to readiness to seek professional help, where the true rate of distress is masked by the fact that women tend to ask more frequently and earlier for professional intervention. European women's readiness to ask for such support comes in part from being seen and seeing themselves as weaker than men, as well as from having a greater readiness to explore relationships and emotions, and from being less ready to repress personal unhappiness. This readiness needs to be seen in its cultural context, in which some central parts of everyday life in Europe have been psychologised – notably motherhood, childhood and adult loving relationships – since the Second World War.[28]

In contrast, psychologisation at this level has not taken place in Asia, and indeed Asian women immigrants in Europe do not refer themselves as often to mental health services as do indigenous women. It is more likely that their daughters will do so, provided they have overcome the greater stigma within their ethnic group concerning mental distress and being seen to be using a mental health service.[29]

Social labelling has been proposed as the third alternative explanation for the higher rate of women as users of mental health services. This assumes a tendency among lay people and professionals to perceive women's reactions to distress as less rational and less conforming with social norms. This goes back to mental health being defined in masculine terms, and its absence in women as a reflection of mental imbalance, although it applies equally to men who express their unhappiness in ways that are socially unacceptable, that is, display mental illness 'symptoms'.

Secondary labelling has been identified in relation to the large number of women who are prescribed minor tranquillisers and become highly dependent on them, only to find themselves labelled as drug addicts. Secondary labelling is often extended to assumptions about the inability of women sufferers to be good at anything. This may at times lead to disastrous results in terms of the removal of children and the severing of ties between them and their mothers.

The emergence of sexual abuse and of anorexia and self-mutilation as women's issues in the second half of the 1980s highlights the depth and severity of what some women in our midst are going through, and the interpretation of what it means to be a woman that some of them have opted for.[30] The generalised effect of labelling applies to men too, in particular in relation to assumed violence.

Jack[31] has proposed that some working-class women internalise a generalised attributional framework that includes low self-esteem and an expectation of being badly treated by others, leading them to repeated suicide attempts as the only autonomous act left to them. He is thus suggesting a link between expectations based on class, gender and psychiatric symptomatology.

A discussion of women in special hospitals, where issues of harm to oneself and others are prominent, is presented in Chapter 4.

The perspective of women users of mental health services

Unlike users of such services from ethnic minorities, women users have been able to express their views in writing, at meetings, and by being active in user groups.[32] Many of the issues they have raised are shared with men users, such as unhappiness with the overuse of medication, and the lack of counselling, work opportunities and decent housing. Women have raised the issue of being physically attacked, as well as sexually harassed and attacked, while in hospital, and of personal belongings being stolen there. They have further suggested that they are not believed when they complain about current or past abuse.[33]

Women users have complained of an overreadiness to hospitalise them and to take away their children, without sufficient provisions being made for them to see their children or to have the support required to continue to look after them when they leave hospital. There are very few facilities for babies to stay with mothers experiencing psychiatric problems, and none for toddlers or school-age children. Women sufferers have expressed a clear preference for female staff while in hospital, a practice that some hospitals have begun to adopt.

Women who are lesbians feel that when their sexual orientation is known, their mental distress is attributed to this preference[34] and that their negative life events are minimised (such as separation from or the death of a partner).

Women as carers

Most of the relatives actually living with and caring for people with mental illness are women, usually mothers or wives. However there is no literature and no European research on this issue (as distinct from the general research on relatives reviewed in

Chapters 2 and 4), while there is a growing body of research on women as carers of sufferers from physical disabilities and dementia.[35] This highlights the fact that despite caring being perceived as an integral component of women's roles and identity (the care of children growing up, one's partner), it is treated as socially peripheral and undesirable when it pertains to looking after people who are disabled. It would therefore seem that the stigma attached to disability is contagious in being attributed to the informal caring role. The newly introduced carers' allowance goes some way towards addressing the inherent negative attitude to informal carers, despite the formal positive attitude.

Men and mental distress

In some feminist literature it is assumed that the reasons leading to mental breakdown in men are different from those experienced by women. This assumption is based on the negation of the right of men to experience unhappiness, to feel inferior, weak, dominated by others or unfulfilled. I would argue that this amounts to denying the humanity of men. Interestingly, attempts to include men in understanding what is happening to women have come in part from feminist family therapists, as well as feminist writers on fatherhood. O'Brien[36] outlines evidence that strongly indicates that men seek much less psychological and psychiatric support for themselves than women, are much less likely to seek such help for family members or to participate in family therapy. In analysing the reasons for these findings, Briscoe proposes three factors:[37]

- Problem recognition: namely that fewer men recognise emotional problems as such when they come across them.
- Expressive differences: men are socialised not to express emotional concern, which is connected to perceived weakness. They accept the social role given to mothers in particular, and to a lesser degree to all women, to be the gatekeepers of emotional reactions to misfortune, and the identifiers of psychological problems.
- Institutional factors: mental health services are structured in a way that makes it more difficult for men who work to attend, and the stigma attached to such attendance may impact on job

promotion prospects (this is based on the erroneous assumption that most women do not work outside their homes).

Furthermore, part of the institutional constraint is the discomfort experienced by both male and female therapists in working with men,[38] reflecting the extent to which therapists too have internalised social norms concerning gender and therapy.

In the process of making a training video, in 1991 I went to one of the most participatory mental health settings in Britain, the Tontine Road Mental Health Project (now renamed the Chesterfield Support Network). There I spent some time talking to the men and women who were members of the large, self-managed users' group. When asked about the topics discussed in a men's group, the young man who acted as the spokesperson of the group mentioned sexuality, violence and alcohol, which he described as 'men's issues'. The topic put forward by list the spokesperson of the women's group in the same centre consisted of loneliness and sexual abuse. These two lists seem to indicate that assumed gender differences have been internalised to a large extent by users too. Yet the sexual abuse of boys, and anorexia, depression and suicide attempts among adolescent and young adult men[39] started to become noticeable in the 1980s. These revelations reflect the similarity in the psychological and social issues that both men and women face in Europe today.

More men are categorised as exhibiting *challenging behaviour*, discussed in Chapter 2 as a category destined to replace psychopathy and inadequate personality in vagueness and stigmatisation, while continuing to be related to socially unacceptable behaviour that is not criminal. The same applies to alcohol and drug abuse. In addition, men dominate as abusers and perpetrators of violent acts, often against women and children. Yet this violence is only infrequently perceived as a sign of mental distress.

The increase in unemployment throughout Europe during the 1980s hit men harder than women, as more full-time jobs disappeared than part-time jobs. In fact the major growth area of jobs has been in part-time jobs, most of which are taken up by women, because of the rather sexist assumption that women do not need a full-time posts, given their responsibilities at home, but that men do need full-time jobs to fulfil their familial obligations.

Evidence of the impact of unemployment on men's physical and mental health accumulated throughout the 1970s and 1980s,[40] demonstrating the irrefutable damage to both types of health, as highlighted in Chapter 5 (where the impact of unemployment on women will be looked at too). Pertaining to mental health, the damage is to a man's identity not only as a breadwinner, but also to his potency as an achiever, given that work – and the power gained through work in European societies – is the main vehicle of achieving social status.

The impact that the dictate to repress softness and vulnerability has had on men's sexuality and mental health should perhaps be made more explicit than it has been so far. The impact of this repression probably also extends to the use of alcohol and drugs as escape measures, allowing the uncomfortable and unexpressed to remain hidden but less bothersome in the short term, while pursuing a macho image.

The increase in attempted suicide and completed suicide among young men during the 1980s is closely related to regional rates of unemployment,[41] the repression of frustration and the blow to unemployed men's social and personal position, as well as to the use of suicide as a 'shock tactic' that fits the stereotypical macho image of men as bold and brave.

The coming out of gay men and women and the greater acceptance of homosexuality and lesbianism in European societies must have liberated a large number of men and women from the burden of leading a hidden and stigmatised life. Yet the socialised guilt and shame must continue to burden many people with a minority sexual orientation, as – at best – this more accepting social attitude is often only skin-deep and very recent. Their sense of guilt, shame and failure, and the fear of AIDS and HIV among gay men, are likely to be expressed in a variety of forms, of which mental distress and illness are two distinct possibilities.

Conceptual innovations concerning gender and mental distress

The focus on gender in relation to mental distress has come from the women's movement and feminist ways of thinking. Linking issues faced by women to their social position and the psychological connotations of this position has enabled us to understand not only the higher rate of mental distress identified among women, but more importantly the socio-psychological base of the definitions of mental health and distress and its centrality to understanding women and working with them. By extension, the same applies to men. Furthermore, the socially desirable definition of mental health has been questioned and found wanting, as it focuses too much on some aspects of our existence while neglecting others, at our peril.

Depression, as a generalised reaction rather than just a clinical category, has been perceived as the mode of women's reaction to their untenable position, in which they are expected to provide care but not to take care of themselves, as well as to compete with men in the world of work. The literature on caring has helped us to understand its ambiguous nature and social position. Women's manifested mental distress has been perceived as an attempt to come to terms with and/or rebel against these impositions, which have included looking as men want women to look, being perfect mothers/daughters/wives.[42]

In a way, the unanswered question is why so many women have not manifested signs of mental distress, and not only why so many women have demonstrated such signs. The answer lies not only in individual circumstances, but in part in the support structures available, which vary by class and ethnicity, degree of social and geographical mobility and emotional ties, and the effect the women's movement had on changing women's and men's perspectives and patterns of relationship. The conceptual aspect expressed in the women's movement has provided us with a partial analysis of why women become mentally distressed, and why they remain psychiatric patients.

Gender-sensitive interventions

Such interventions were creatively invented in relation to women, and less so in relation to men. This has been the case because interventions for to women were developed in conjunction with the development of the women's movement, whereas no successful parallel movement has been developed for and by men.

The women's movement has also provided us with an innovative intervention strategy in its focus on the value of sharing subjective experiences, discussing emotions, providing mutual support and flattening hierarchies, and accepting weaknesses as both part of human nature and the result of social injustice. Above all it has given women pride in what they are, and with it the right to take care of themselves.

A striking example of such a difference can be observed in a poor suburb of Naples, where a public sector mental health service for women is run side by side with a service for men. The services are run by two consultant psychiatrists, who happen to be partners in their private lives too. Situated on the same floor, the women's service rooms are well decorated. The service offers a gender-sensitive approach, which includes individual and group counselling, a minimal use of medication, and a number of work projects and recreation. The men's service is located in run-down rooms, and provides a traditional assessment and medication-dominated service. No work projects, no recreation opportunities and hardly any counselling seem to be on offer.

Gender-sensitivity at the intervention facet begins with attention to *purchasing*. Williams *et al*.[43] have researched the issue and published an intelligent and imaginative booklet entitled *Purchasing Effective Mental Health Services for Women: A Framework for Action*. They outline what women currently receive in the way of mental health services, the unacknowledged causes of women's distress, and what women do and do not want from services and service providers. The booklet includes examples, mostly drawn from not-for-profit services, and demonstrates the value of adopting a participatory stance in purchasing services.

Thus the booklet reflects that the particular style developed by the women's movement, namely the focus on *participation* and flattening the hierarchy – typical of the new social movements of the 1960s and 1970s, including the women's movement – happens also to be a most useful tool in enabling people to rebuild threatened identities, by empowering them individually while connecting them to a supportive network that offers solidarity as a bonus.

Consciousness raising through this form of groupwork has been further developed into the *self-directed groupwork* model.[44] A variety of self-directed groupwork forms have been utilised in projects focusing on mental distress issues for women, such as the Neighbourhood Project and the Battersea Project in the 1970s, the White City Women in Mental Health Project and the Nottingham groups of women whose children were abused in the 1980s, and the Trieste Women's Space in the 1990s.[45]

The Trieste Women's Space is now occupying an ex-mental health building. It is run by a joint management committee of women mental health professionals, women service users and 'ordinary' women from the city, and has been functioning since 1992. Women's Space activities have included a poetry festival, theatre productions, demonstrations for peace in former Yugoslavia (Trieste borders with Slovenia and Croatia), side by side with group discussions on mental distress issues, and make-up and flower arranging courses.

The London Women's Therapy Centre represents another outcome of the women's movement, this time influenced more by North American developments. The centre is run as a not-for-profit service. It provides psychoanalytically oriented psychotherapy in which the difficulties experienced by women due to their social position and the critique of orthodox psychoanalysis have been taken into account. In addition it provides training courses for women workers in mental health services.

Since the beginning of the 1980s some family therapists have been engaged in addressing the major issues coming out of feminist understanding and beliefs within their practice. Such issues include taking account of power relations in the family and in educational and work settings, of handling sexual abuse as a gender issue (among its other ramifications), tackling resistance to such a perspective among colleagues, and working with men in a way that is gender-sensitive towards them too, and not only towards their women partners.[46] In working with men there are fewer innovations. The suggestion that action-related therapy is likely to appeal more to men is questioned on the ground that it in fact fosters existing stereotypes about the lower status of emotions and reflective discussions. Minuchin's 'executive-style' in family therapy sessions is likewise doubted.[47]

Barry Mason and Ed Mason have proposed the use of a gender-neutral approach, defined as 'challenging belief systems without taking sides'.[48] Following this method, issues raised by one partner are reflected to the other partner in than attempt to raise consciousness over gender differences while being evenhanded. This has been criticised as being gender-blind.

All too often women receive support only from the more traditional mainstream services. Traditional work with women and men continues in outpatient clinics, psychiatric hospitals and psychiatric wards in general hospitals, as well as in community mental health centres, child guidance clinics and social services departments, and above all by the first professional port of call, the GP.

While some mental health centres recognise the importance of gender issues and enable women (though rarely men) to get together in a group side by side with individual work, this does not extend to most mainstream services. Most interventions consist of prescribing medication in a sympathetic way. Most services consider women as mothers only, and pay no attention to their other needs, wishes or social roles. Fifteen years after the publication of the work of Brown and Harris on the social origin of depression,[49] which demonstrated the importance of a psychosocial approach to women suffering from depression, the British Royal College of Psychiatrists' latest campaign on depression still makes no mention of issues to do with gender. Likewise a recent book by two eminent women professionals on counselling in primary care omits gender, female and male, from consideration.[50] It is therefore perhaps unsurprising that separatist services and groups continue to be cherished and that more of such services are desired by women. This particularly true of survivors of sexual abuse, but not only.

A small number of services pay combined attention to issues of ethnicity and gender. For example the Southall Black Sisters, a highly politicised group of young, well-educated Asian women, now provides a service for Asian women suffering from mental illness and domestic violence. Shanti, in South London, works with Afro-Caribbean women suffering from mental health problems, using individual and groupwork methods. Throughout Europe there are many informal, not-for-profit, small-scale organisations that offer women advice, advocacy and counselling, without necessarily being defined as mental health services. Often these concentrate on women refugees or recent immigrants (for example in Berlin, Copenhagen, Naples and Turin). There are also a number of mutual support groups for women suffering from specific distresses (anorexia, minor tranquillisers, survivors of sexual abuse).

Are separatist services the only way forward? Why did women

professionals in the Trieste mental health services, who for many years resisted separatist services, opt in 1992 for an experimental women's space? In part, their former reluctance came out of a belief in the universal view of mental distress, combined with the wish to provide an equitable service across the gender divide. To provide a separatist service is to accept the limitations of the universalist model, if not its failure. In part, this general state of affairs is due to continued belief in the somatic origin of mental illness, which does not necessitate consideration of psychosocial factors. It also partly reflect, the inherent difficulty of working on issues that are greatly influenced by *structural factors* through means that are mainly located at the individual level, or at most at the small group level, while their remedy lies in changes affecting the political and ideological level of the whole society.

Thus the justified glow of the innovative, empathic and interesting work outlined above should not blind us to what it cannot achieve.

4
Long-term Users of Mental Health Services

Definitions and their significance for stakeholders

The terms 'long-term' and 'continuing/continued' clients came into use in the 1980s, replacing the term 'chronic'. As suggested in Chapter 2, the latter was perceived as negatively judgemental and as predetermining the likelihood of a mental health service user remaining seriously distressed forever.

While in Europe the two terms are still in intermittent use, in the 1980s in North America terms such as the 'seriously and critically ill' or 'severely and persistently mentally ill' were brought into use. The different terms encapsulate differences in value judgements concerning severity, disability, chronicity, ability, origins of mental illness, the likelihood of cure and the desirable forms of care.

None of these terms should be confused with 'long stay', coined in the 1970s and denoting people who are hospitalised for more then two years, in comparison with 'short stay', that is, those remaining in hospital for less than two years. Within 'long stay' a further distinction was made between the 'old long stay' and the 'new old stay', namely between those staying for more then five years and deemed old in age, and those staying for less then five years and younger in age.[1] The latter distinction was made to express the surprise that, after the introduction of psychotropic drugs, a number of young people in their twenties did not recover and seemed to require more than the short admissions that were possible in acute units in general hospitals, as well as a way of writing-off the 'old long stay' as being beyond reach of rehabilitative intervention.

The recognition and acceptance by professionals that people suffering from some forms of mental illness require long-term support, rather than brief support that can be terminated without harmful effects, became prominent in the late 1970s too. This coincided with the receding of the euphoria created by the introduction of psychotropic drugs and the evaporation of claims as to their effectiveness. According to Warner[2] about a third of all people suffering from schizophrenia improved considerably with the use of the new drugs; another third improved marginally; and the condition of the remaining third worsened as a direct result of using the drugs. Comparable figures have been suggested for depression and manic-depressive illness.

Faced with the relative lack of cure through the use of medication for people suffering from major mental illness categories, it became imperative to understand the reasons for this state of affairs and to explain it within professional circles first. Relatives and users required explanations too, as did politicians, who formally give the social mandate to mental health professionals.

Professional stakeholders' views

Psychiatrists

The majority of European psychiatrists, starting from the viewpoint that mental illness is a biological disturbance, came to the conclusion that the main reason for the lack of cure is the depth of the biological defect. Concepts such as 'positive' symptoms (florid), 'negative' symptoms (social disfunctioning and apathy) and 'primary' and 'secondary' handicaps were invented in the attempt to make sense of the evidence of partial improvements and the reoccurrence of distressing and socially unacceptable behaviour. The impact of the services and structures in which people were treated was perceived as part of the 'secondary' handicaps. The possibility of psychological and social aetiology underlying such an illness was seen as unconvincing.

Thus Wing and Furlong[3] define this client group as 'mentally disordered adults, in addition to those with mental handicap and dementia, who are highly dependent on others and have a high all round need for care which had hitherto been equated with a need for long term residence in hospital'.

Since the 1940s a minority of psychiatrists have considered that both the impact of the institutional framework and the psychosocial environment in which people live prior to and after hospitalisation are of central significance in the lead-up to mental illness and in maintaining its reappearance, as exemplified in the work of Maxwell Jones.[4] Levander,[5] working in Sweden, suggested that people with long-term mental distress, originally of a psychotic nature and living mainly in the community, are not actually lost between the institutions, but rather *absorbed* within psychiatry in a way that tends to preserve them in their chronic patient role. Psychiatric services often become the core of their lives, their main provider, and the location of their social network.

A framework focusing on a psychoanalytical perspective of psychosis was developed in France during the 1960s and 1970s, which has influenced some public sector services.[6] It is based on the belief that by the application of psychoanalytical methods it is possible to reverse the process of chronicity and deterioration among people suffering from these illnesses.

Basaglia's, Piro's and Rotelli's approach,[7] exemplifying Italian psychiatric reform, differed from the perspectives just outlined above in differentiating the initial reasons for becoming mentally ill from the reasons for remaining in this category. They proposed that either biological, psychological or social reasons – or a combination of all three – could lie behind the initial eruption of mental illness, but that its perpetuation is due primarily to social segregation. Within this framework chronicity is the direct result of segregation, isolation, social devaluing and not being given the opportunity to reenter ordinary social interaction. Furthermore professionals have colluded with ruling groups to segregate people suffering from mental illness, to prevent them from being visible, and to present their fate as a fate to be avoided by those entertaining non-conforming possibilities.

A fourth strand is provided by those who focus on rehabilitation. As De Plato has suggested,[8] rehabilitation has be come a replacement for cure among professionals who believe in the circularity of the interaction between the person and the environment, and biological and social factors (interestingly he does not mention the psychological aspect). Benedetto Saraceno, currently president of the international Social Rehabilitation Association, simply states that rehabilitation is a practice without a theory,[9] referring to our current hazy state of knowledge.

Thus a wide range of attempts to understand and explain the

existence of people in need of long-term support exists within psychiatry itself.

Nurses

Nurses, the largest professional group within mental health services in most countries (less so in Greece, Portugal and Slovenia), do not seem to have a view of their own on these issues. Most of them accept the need for long-term support as they have internalised the view that the illness is continually lurking in the wings. Community Psychiatric Nurses (CPNs), a new branch of nursing developed in the late 1970s specifically to work in a non-hospital setting, are split between those who wish to work with people with long-term mental health problems, and those who prefer to work with people experiencing short-term mental distress.

Lynne, an experienced nurse working in a CPN team in a seaside English town, told me that she did not wish to work 'upstairs' (where the team working with continued care clients was located) as *'it smells of death* to work with these people'. Instead she was taking a counselling course, is in psychoanalytic psychotherapy, and saw her future as a counsellor.

Her colleague Helen, who was working upstairs, told me that she was finding it difficult to work with so many nurses who disliked being near people with long-term mental illness. She elaborated by saying that they gave her the feeling that there was nothing to be done, whereas she felt that much could be done to improve the lives of continued care clients by nurses who care. All the examples she gave were to do with the social and psychological aspects of living, even though she was responsible for administering medication and supporting the people taking it. In a similar vein, Italian nurses have spoken about the psychological and social support they provide to continued care clients as the most satisfactory part of their work.[10] The implications of these approaches will be looked at in Chapter 7.

It would therefore appear that, without formally discarding the biological and more somatic aspects of mental illness, informally members of the new branches of psychiatric nursing focus more on non-biological aspects in their quest for professional success and satisfaction.

Psychologists

Psychologists represent a numerically small group in all European countries, but they are influential in terms of their impact on understanding and explaining, in part due to the way psychology evolved as an academic and research discipline before becoming an applied discipline.

Most European psychologists side with psychosocial reasoning for the first appearance of mental illness.[11] Therefore they tend to view the presenting crisis as the tip of an iceberg, where the iceberg is to do with close interpersonal relationships, intrapsychological conflicts or faulty learning habits. Continuing support is required to enable the person to change feelings, perceptions and behaviours. Sinason's application of Klein's psychoanalytic tradition to working with people suffering from learning difficulties, sexual abuse and psychotic episodes reflects one strand of such an approach in its recent form.[12]

Behaviourists tend to opt for time-limited focused intervention rather than unlimited support. This relates to the body of research that illustrates how people's ability to change usually comes in short bursts, and that continued intervention only decreases the level of motivation and engagement in the change process.

However psychologists of all schools working within residential settings seem to have accepted the need for prolonged and continuous support, punctuated by periodical reviews and the replanning of individual and group objectives. This could be due to recognition of the depth of the vulnerability of the person, caused by either the illness and/or the damage inflicted by years of institutionalisation, to which the majority of people in residential settings have been subjected.

Psychologists adhering to the normalisation and social role valorisation approach seem to have crossed the boundary between the psychological and the social, leaving the biological behind.[13]

Social workers

Social workers have been trained to accept the priority of psychological and social factors in the lives of their clients, but also that of assumed vulnerability, together with a potential for improvement in the future.[14] Such vulnerability does not rule out biological factors and the interaction between different factors. The acceptance of vulnerability and the focus on future potential emphasise the long-term nature of the necessary support and fragility of the person and/or their environment. At the same time social workers assume that long-term support acts as a *preventive measure* against a small-scale crisis developing into a large-scale disaster. Therefore social workers assume the need for long-term support without having to judge the issue of failure to cure and its significance. In fact the majority of social workers find it difficult to operate within short-term frameworks.[15]

Thus the social work perspective is multilayered while appearing to be deceptively simple.

The perspectives of indirect and direct service users

Relatives

Relatives assume that major mental illnesses are a life-long condition, like a chronic physical illness (for example multiple sclerosis). They suggest that psychotropic drugs might allow short or prolonged periods of remission, but do not anticipate a cure. Therefore they expect the related services to support family members suffering from major mental illnesses on a continuous basis, and to extend that support to them if required.[16] Many of them are likely to see hospitals as the best and safest medical sites for intervention. Some of their definitional dilemmas are summarised in the following quotation of a relative's view:

> what I was saying about A. that I believe her condition isn't curable with a strictly logical approach. In some sense her perception of the world is more real than that of the doctors'. She can actually see, she has got visions of angles, and devils and things which in a way are floating around and which in a way are sort of governing our lives, whether we know it or not. Its just that she is unabalanced, unable to switch it off.[17]

Users

Users vary in their views on the impact of major mental illnesses. Those active in the European Users Network (which is described below in this chapter in the section on user-led initiatives) believe that the illness is a reaction to an untenable position created by others and therefore curable in the sense of either changing the situation or moving away from the people who have created it, while the person receives psychological and social support. For them, traditional psychiatric intervention has led to further oppression and perpetuation of the untenable situation.[18] They are also sceptical of formal definitions that leave out subjective experiences and suffering, substituting them for impersonal categorisation.

Others, such as members of Voices (the users' group that forms part of the British National Schizophrenia Fellowship) follow the beliefs of relatives, outlined above.

The impact of the rediscovery of the continued care client

This rediscovery has been looked at in terms of its conceptual framework in Chapter 2. The reasons for and the sources of the rediscovery go some way towards accounting for its impact:[19]

- scandals concerning conditions of hospitalisation (in the 1950s);
- rethinking by some professionals, critical of the traditional system and of traditional professional attitudes and interventions (since the 1940s, but especially in the 1960s and 1980s), who have come to reject the psychiatric hospital as a useful location for psychiatric intervention.
- largely positive outcomes to resettlement and rehabilitation programmes in and out of hospitals (since the 1940s, beginning with the therapeutic communities);
- government interest in reducing public spending and readiness to reformulate policies and restructure mental health systems (beginning in the United States in the late 1960s, in Britain at the beginning of the 1980s, and in Italy in the late 1980s).
- the emergence of more vocal relatives' groups (since the 1970s in the United States, the 1980s in Britain and Italy);
- the emergence of more vocal users' groups (since the 1970s in the United States, The Netherlands, Finland and Sweden, the 1980s in Britain and Italy).

The new, more multifaceted, varied and open-ended construct of the continued care client does not lend itself to neat definitions, including diagnostic categorisation, nor to neat working models.

The readiness to accept variability *within* a group of continued care clients implies that it is more up to individual workers and clients to read what they want into the construct (which is mediated by their interpretation of a given situation and personal circumstances). Such a reading would evolve out of specific encounters and relationships between workers and clients. It is especially up to teams of professionals to develop ways of thinking, relating, and intervening that allow and encourage continued care clients to be seen as multidimensional human beings, rather then as the one-dimensional category – 'the mentally ill' – they were presumed to be.

When I met Jean for the first time she was active in a new users' pressure group, and had been a client of mental health services for about ten years. She seemed shy, but effective and well organised. Later we were both members of a user–worker organisation that was critical of the psychiatric establishment, and she was one of the most articulate members of the group. I noticed that she did not socialise much with either users or workers, but developed more friendly relations with one member of the group who was in an ambiguous position, and visited her at home a couple of times.

Jean began to look unwell, developed an allergy on her hands, and was not around for a couple of months. One day I went to visit a psychiatric hospital and saw her in the grounds. She looked at me as if she did not recognise me, and I did not attempt to approach her. She had put on a lot of weight, and her gaze was vacant. I asked one of the workers about her, who replied that she would be fine soon, but that when she exploded everyone was terrified.

When I saw her next at the meetings of the group she had lost weight and was her active self again. I heard that she was in psychotherapy and was engaged in work experience with a voluntary organisation. After a couple of months she announced that she was leaving the group, and would like to concentrate on activities that had nothing to do with mental distress.

Jean indeed left the group, worked towards a postgraduate qualification in a helping profession, and terminated the few personal contacts she had in the group. Jean is not 'representative' of continued care clients, in part because she has moved from being a user to being a worker. If she is continuing to be in psychotherapy, then she is now occupying *both* roles. Who is 'representative' of this client group? The people who attend smoky day centres for the rest of their lives? The people who return for short admissions every six months? The people who end up in special hospitals? Those who commit suicide? The very few who commit homicide? Or those who become workers again, advocates, writers, parents, sit on management committees? *All* are long-term users of mental health services, and Jean could have become any one of them, with a slight twist of events, different actors, or lack of luck.

Size

The issue of size depends on the definition applied to mental distress. As each of the definitions spans across diagnostic categories, refers to people mostly living in the community, and to a state of being, it is unsurprising that precise numbers are difficult to come by. In countries where the majority of people with mental illness are hospitalised for prolonged periods, the inpatient figure provides a reasonable, but insufficient, indicator of the size of this group. In such countries it is likely that a number of people in need of long-term support but living in the community are not known to the services, as they do not appear in any statistics. Thus in Greece, out of 97 00 000 inhabitants 6211 were inpatients in 1990; only 1591 people appeared to be attending rehabilitation centres, group homes and day centres.[20] In Slovenia, with 25 00 000 inhabitants, 10 000 were hospitalised in 1993;[21] no figures exist for people in need of long-term support who are living in the community, primarily because there are virtually no specific services catering for them.

In contrast, most Western European countries have a variety of community services where long-term users can be located (such as outpatient clinics, day centres, sheltered housing, sheltered workshops, community mental health centres), apart from places in psychiatric hospitals and psychiatric wards in general hospitals. Yet the availability of services in the community does not seem to make it any easier to calculate a figure with confidence. For example a recent British official publication (*Health of the Nation*, February 1994) suggests that 250 000 people are suffering from schizophrenia in Britain out of a general population of 57 000 000), whereas Grove[22] has suggested that long-term users consist of the 100000 people recently resettled from hospitals into the community, plus those currently in hospital for repeated admission (about 40 000–50 000 people), or a total of 150000 out of a population of 57 million.

Table 4.1 describes the situation in the Swedish outpatients services.

To estimate the size of the Swedish continued care client population we need to add the figures of those suffering from psychosis, personality disorder and some of those in the substance abuse category. We still do not know how many in the 'other' category may require long-term attention.

Who are the service users?

The inpatients subgroup

This group includes more women, more people over 65 (the 'old long stay') and more people in the 25–44 age group (the

Table 4.1 Estimate of psychiatric outpatients with different diagnoses and number of visits in 1991 (based on a one-day nationwide survey)

Diagnosis	Survey estimated No.			Pat. per no. of visits
	per year		100 000	per year
Neurotic	4.482	68.500	810	822.000
Personality disorder	1.310	6.000	80	96.000
Psychosis	3.307	26.500	310	530.000
Substance abuse*	700.000	19.000	220	171.000
Other	686.000	18.000	220	131.000
Total	10.485	138.800	1.640	1.750.600

*Alcohol and drug abuse, when this is the primary diagnosis.
Source: U. Brinck, 'Psychiatric care and social support for the long-term mentally disturbed in Sweden', *International Journal of Social Psychiatry*, vol. 40, no. 4 (1994).

'new long stay') than either below 25 or between 44 and 65. Numerically more older people than young people suffer from long-term mental distress. Yet Ciompi has systematically demonstrated that, with the exception of dementia in the over-85 age group, most psychiatric illness categories diminish in frequency and prevalence, as well as in symptomatology.[23] Ethnic composition and gender have been looked at in Chapter 3.

We know little about the non-psychiatric characteristics of this group, as the individualised files of most psychiatric services do not record attempts to get to know the patient as a person. The files reflect the fact that people are approached as objects of inquiry and intervention, and their wishes, strengths and individuality are not noted. When people in this category are encouraged to talk about their lives and their understanding of it, a different picture emerges – of people with a past and a future.[24]

The years spent in hospital do not figure at all in the life stories told by them, even though for most of them these years represent a large part of their chronological life. This is not due to any lack of memory or direct repression. It is more likely to be the result of the recognition that so little happened over these years in terms of events, in particular little that was personal, and that these years represent a personal failure that the person would rather not dwell upon.

Since the beginning of the 1990s I have visited psychiatric hospitals in Britain, Czechoslovakia, Greece, Holland, Hungary, Portugal, Russia, Slovenia and Ukraine, as well as psychiatric wards in general hospitals in these countries and in Italy. Life in all of them is remarkably similar, even if the physical conditions are not and the range of facilities within the hospitals differ. Life in hospital continues to be regimented, lacking in privacy, in choice, in encouraging initiative and networking among the residents. It fosters impersonal relationships between residents and workers and provides a boring daily routine, where the highlights of the day consist mainly of mealtime and a smoke.

Underlying this impoverished life style are three assumptions:

- Asylum is about a full retreat from ordinary living, to the point of total passivity and compliance.

- People assumed to be ill are also supposed to be unable to enjoy themselves (Christmas parties are the exception, at which they are ordered to enjoy themselves) and should not be 'over-stimulated' – that is, given opportunities to enjoy themselves. Alternatively this may be a reflection of the view that hospitalisation should not be enjoyed, as this would foster dependency and further retreat from ordinary responsibilities.
- The task of getting better does not consist of more than obeying the doctor's orders and taking the prescribed medication on time.

Leros hospital, on the Greek island with the same name, has become a 'cause celebre' of a place, infamous for the lack of dignity accorded to its inmates.[25] The site was initially an Italian naval base (built before the Second World War), and then became a psychiatric hospital on an island to which political prisoners were exiled during the military rule of Greece, and where orphans of murdered political opponents were adopted by local families. I was in Leros in 1993, nine years after the initiative sponsored by the European Community began in 1984 (described in Chapter 1). Most wards still lacked showers, toilets with seats, drinking water between 6.00 p.m. and 8.00 a.m., wardrobes, warm blankets, good quality mattresses, wards with less than twenty people, window curtains, curtains between beds to delineate privacy, laid tables at mealtime with enough cups per person, pictures on the walls, let alone recreational areas, indoor activities, rehabilitation facilities and sheltered work schemes. A number of people walked barefoot – it was pointed out to me that there was a cupboard full of shoes, but these were not in use as the person responsible for the inventory would need to replace any lost pairs.

Yet this was an improvement on the previous situation, in which the majority of patients were kept naked and food was distributed by means of putting it in a single bucket in the middle of a large room, in which patients also urinated and left their faeces (there were no toilets).

The effect of this utter lack of dignity was well reflected in a rather unexpected incident that I happened to observe. I arrived in a ward – infamous in the past because patients had been kept naked there – when one of the patients had just choked to death. The staff were trying desperately to revive him, but *all* the other inpatients *moved neither towards him nor away from him*. They seemed not to have taken it in that something out of the ordinary was happening, and that it was happening to one of them.

This level of numbness, of being cut off from the world of the living, of being dead psychologically and socially, though not physically, is the direct result of living for years in a repressive and abusive regime.

This state of affairs cannot be attributed to the patients' mental illness and/or mental handicap. Just a few hundred metres on the outside perimeter of the hospital there was a small house in which ten people taken out of this ward had been living for the past two years. There they lived three to a bedroom, with ordinary, warm furnishings and attention. They were responding positively to this dramatic change: some had begun to be able to feed themselves with the use of cutlery, after years of using only their hands and having to fight to get food from the communal bucket. Some had begun to use words to express themselves, having ceased to speak in the years they had spent in the ward.

Little is known in terms of follow-up of non-resettled inpatients. McCreadie and McCannell[26] have carried out a survey of Scottish inpatients, defined as 'the new chronic inpatients', covering 14 psychiatric hospitals and two psychiatric units in general hospitals that serve 56 per cent of the Scottish population. Of the 571 who were so defined in 1982, 71 per cent remained inpatients in 1984. In 1987, at the end of the five-year follow-up study, 22 per cent of the initial group had died and 50 per cent were still inpatients. Sixty-five per cent of the deaths had been caused by bronchopneumonia or heart disease, suicide accounted for 6 per cent.

Of the 285 people remaining in hospital, less than half of the 1982 figure were in a closed ward, fewer were detained, a somewhat larger number were on parole, and about the same number were on a long-stay or rehabilitation ward. According to the researchers, 38 per cent of the 1984 group and 37 per cent of the 1987 cohort did not need to stay in hospital for psychiatric treatment purposes, as their rehabilitation scores showed a significant improvement in the scales of dependency, activity, isolation and symptoms. Most of the them tended to fall into the younger, 'new long stay' subgroup.

Living in a special hospital

All European countries have specialised facilities for people suffering from mental illness and deemed dangerous. A sizeable proportion of these inpatients have not committed an offence. In the early 1990s the number of people residing in special hospitals in Britain and Italy, two countries with a comparable population size (57 million and 55 million respectively) were 1700 and 1600 respectively.[27] These special hospitals are run as a separate health authority. Similarly there is a special intermediary structure between prisons and ordinary psychiatric hospitals in Holland and a 'prison prevention' structure in France.[28]

Interestingly there is no correlation between the number of people in these specialised settings and the overall number of prisoners in each European country. Britain heads the list of the number of imprisoned people, while Italy occupies the fourth place from the bottom.[29] This is particularly relevant data, given that Italy:

- has closed more psychiatric hospitals than Britain has so far;
- has a poorer public welfare system, yet a lower number of homeless people;
- and, as mentioned in Chapter 2, shows no fear of the new long stay; yet neither does it show the zeal to reincarcerate those ex-patients who refuse to take their medication regularly that has been demonstrated in Britain recently.

Bearing in mind the wish to prevent harm to others and self-harm, we need to ask whether a separate structure for people who have committed offences and suffer from mental distress is the best solution? Would a good prison psychiatric service suffice? Is a special structure more humane than prison? These are just some of the questions that are usually not asked, as the established professional and political wisdom is that a medical setting is always an improvement on a penal setting. In terms of treating people suffering from mental illness, it might be preferable for them go to prison for an offence they admit committing, even if carried out while unwell, and carry the responsibility for their actions in the way that everybody else does, as long as they also receive good psychiatric care. At the same time it is true that prison regimes are notoriously cruel and undignified, and being there may serve to increase the level of mental distress already experienced.

A recent study on women on remand (that is, awaiting trial) in a London prison found that the medical officer of the prison tended to diagnose mental illness as a way of ensuring that women would be referred to psychiatric hospitals, reflecting the view that prison was the wrong place for these women. Psychiatrists coming from the outside to carry out assessments for the courts diagnosed mental illness less often, and less often diagnosed illness of a degree that required hospitalisation.[30]

Most of the women diagnosed as suffering psychosis had committed minor offences, for which they were unlikely to receive a prison sentence. Thus their remand in prison (on average they waited for three weeks to be seen by a psychiatrist) was unnecessary from the safety angle, as well as from the perspective of their mental health, and can be seen as an infringement of their citizens' rights. From the assessments it would seem that the psychiatrists could not suggest alternatives to hospitalisation.

Men assessed as part of court diversion schemes were found to be suffering from psychosis (mainly schizophrenia), homelessness and poor physical health.[31] These studies cannot tell us whether people were homeless first and mentally distressed second, or vice versa. They do indicate that these people, men and women, had extremely deprived backgrounds – materially, socially and emotionally – at the time they were remanded. The findings outline the lack of alternatives to prison or hospital, and the lack of imagination of the professionals in not having the vision to propose such alternatives.

In Britain the physical conditions and staffing levels (mainly unqualified workers) in special hospitals are better than in a number of 'ordinary' psychiatric hospitals, unlike the situation in parallel Italian institutions. Nevertheless special hospitals are prisons and places of known brutality, by both inmates and staff. While only a minority of the staff are known to be maltreating the residents, the number of such incidents has periodically led to public scandals and the setting up of inquiry committees.[32]

There are fewer women in these establishments than men, yet often they are perceived as suffering from a more severe state of psychiatric disturbance, accompanied by self-harm. Women workers and women researchers interested in this group have emphasised that the brutalising environment of the special hospital is harmful to women, and have cast scorn on the proposal for mixed male and female wards as an attempt to use women for the purpose of resocialising men, many of whom have a history of sexual violence.[33] Useful work is being carried out by voluntary groups in Britain, such as WISH (Women In Special Hospitals), which offers advice, counselling and advocacy. Some members of WISH are ex-patients of the special hospitals.

How do women experience the special hospitals? Mary was 22 when she found herself in a special hospital. She was there because she had a history of committing assaults and was accused of arson. Her record does not tell us that she was of mixed race, adopted by a single woman from a white, upper-middle-class background, and that she had failed to live up to the adopting mother's expectations as an adolescent and a young woman. Depression and self-harm represented the other side of the coin.

She hated the special hospital at first: not only being in prison, but being with so many disturbed and distressed people, and with men she was afraid of. Mary's dislike of the place grew when the staff indicated that certain privileges could be given only if she socialised with these men.

A number of self-harm attempts followed. Mary was offered counselling by the psychologist (a woman) and was befriended by one of the older women in her ward. She also worked, and studied for exams. Mary became aware of her lesbian tendencies and was frightened of them. Yet when she managed to accept that this was her sexual orientation she calmed down.

After eleven years in the special hospital Mary left, first to live in a hostel and then in a group home. When I met her she was working for WISH in a part-time capacity, and told her story with great poise and confidence to an audience of more than one hundred people:

You've no control here but you've no control on the outside either. I've been back here twice. I'm never prepared for the outside. I'm on my way back out again and I've got to go back to a place I dread and hate to get out of here. There's nowhere else. A hostel's too big a step. I've been here too long. When you've been here so long you become institutionalised, and you've got no freedom, you're told what to do and treated like a child. They take hold of your life, when you leave here you just can't cope with the freedom you've got.[34]

Coming out of a special hospital in Britain depends not only on an improvement in mental health but on whether another facility is ready to accept that person. People can be discharged on parole with specific conditions to the probation service or social services, and can be recalled during the period of parole. It is very difficult to find an alternative place in an ordinary psychiatric hospital or in the community for this subgroup, as they come with an aura of fear of violence. Existing mental health teams in the community do not see it as their remit to work with this group. In Italy a person enters a special hospital for a recommended minimum stay, after which a review is held to decide whether the person could be discharged. Community mental health services can be responsible for parole supervision. Some community health centres have been successful in both working with discharged patients and preventing committal to a special hospital through the process of psychiatric opinion and by undertaking to work with them in the community.[35]

Secure units exist now in Britain as wards in both psychiatric and general hospitals. They are the favoured British solution to those who suffer from a mental illness and are likely to harm others. It is difficult to see how they differ from special hospitals, apart from their size. They do not exist in Italy.

Living in the community

McCreadie and McCannell's Scottish study (see reference 24) provides information about the 28 per cent of people who were discharged (165 people) by 1987. Of these 38 per cent were living with relatives, 30 per cent on their own and 14 per cent in group homes. Very few were in open employment. Information was lacking for the 37 per cent who did not remain in contact with the services.

A 1991 survey of 500 people who use the services of local Mind branches (Mind is the largest British not-for-profit mental health organisation), of whom 100 were described as continued care clients, indicates that:[36]

- They are primarily poor people living on meagre welfare benefits.
- They are mostly men.
- They have been service users for more than ten years.
- They have not had paid employment for a long time.
- They often do not engage in any activity other than those on offer in a day centre.
- Only a minority attend a day centre, a number of whom do not find such centres to be of interest.
- Most of them have no close contact with their families.
- They tend to be single.
- They have no children.
- They live in sheltered accommodation due to lack of choice.
- They have no hobbies and rarely go out.
- Some have friends, often other people who have also suffered from mental illness.
- Most of them do not exhibit overt symptomatology, but look and act as depressed people.

It would thus seem that these people live the life of poor, isolated people in the community. Resettled people from the long-stay wards of both British and Italian psychiatric hospitals tend to live in staff-supported group homes and attend day centres regularly. Most of them find this new way of life more satisfactory than hospital life in terms of privacy, living conditions, choice, access to communal facilities and to people and places they knew in their past.[37] Yet only a few of them have regular contact with specific people in the community who are not service providers.

I suggested above that the existence of a younger group, often referred to as the 'new long stay', has come as a surprise to professionals and led to an examination of the reasons for its coming into being. Looking at the life-style of this subgroup in the community, especially in comparison with that of the resettled 'long-stay' subgroup, it would seem that they:[38]

- Have a higher rate of repeated admission to psychiatric wards in general hospitals.
- Are likely to be of no fixed abode (that is, without a home, even if they have a bed to sleep in at night).
- Drift into alcohol and drug misuse.
- Have frequent quarrels with relatives and other people they come in contact with.
- Sporadically attend day facilities and outpatient appointments.
- Repeatedly fail rehabilitation attempts in terms of vocational training or placements, or educational courses, despite good intellectual ability and reasonable scholastic achievements.
- Have a tendency to stop taking their medication when they feel better.

There is also a much greater representation of young men in this group than of women, and of black young men in particular.

Most of these young people have been diagnosed as suffering from schizophrenia or personality disorder. Some have been diagnosed as suffering from manic-depressive illness or eating disorders. In many cases self-harm has been attempted. Danish researchers[39] have found that, of 9156 people admitted for the first time over a period of seventeen years (between April 1970 to December 1987) and diagnosed as suffering from schizophrenia, suicide accounted for 50 per cent of reported deaths in men and 35 per cent in women. Only in few cases was harm towards others an issue.

So far there has been no worthwhile research attempting to provide an understanding of these clients' own perspectives, and/or the interaction between them and service providers, between them and their relatives, and between the relatives and the providers. The following is therefore no more than a speculative attempt to make sense of what we know or can infer about this group.

The overarching sense here is of an underlying rage at being misplaced and misunderstood, a rage that cannot be expressed openly, of a person with a promise that was taken away at some point during adolescence or young adulthood from a person who was unable to communicate meaningfully, or felt that he or she had noone with whom to communicate satisfactorily. Being male and an adolescent raises the need to resolve issues of the identity, potency, achievement and competitiveness of someone who is not sure that he can get there, but who needs desperately to demonstrate to himself and others that he can.

Being black is an additional factor, which highlights constraints on opportunities, the impact of being constantly discriminated against, and the impact of internalised expectations of sexual potency and making a place for oneself in the world against all odds in a spectacular way (precisely because the ordinary, non-spectacular ways are less available and less enticing).

While the first breakdown is an expression of all of the above, the reactions to it are crucial in determining whether this event is the beginning of a career as a psychiatric patient or of finding more positive solutions to the issue of identity, potency and place within society.

Some evidence supporting this line of thinking is demonstrated in a study carried out in Birmingham in 1990 by Birchwood et al.,[40] who compared Asian, Afro-Caribbean and white patients in a follow-up after the first admission episode in which schizophrenia was diagnosed. The follow-up illustrated that the Asian group had the lowest relapse rate (16 per cent) followed by whites (30 per cent) and Afro-Caribbeans (49 per cent). In explaining the differences, the authors suggest that speed of access to care, living with a family, and employment opportunities have been more available to the Asian group.

Risk of violence

The issue of the degree of risk of violence – either towards others or oneself – looms large in the media coverage of this group, but less so in the professional literature. Recent British data shows that out of the 250 000 people whom the government suggests are continued care clients, 34 killed another person in the 1991–94 period (as reported by the Royal College of Psychiatrists, *Independent*, 18 August 1994, p. 6), a figure that does *not* represent an increase over the previous three years. One thousand people were murdered in Britain during the same period (that is 966 were killed by people who were not categorised as continued care clients, or as suffering from mental illness). In Italy during the first ten years of the reform (1978–88), no increase in the number of homicides by (or suicide of) people known to suffer from mental illness was reported, or in other European countries for the same period.

Nevertheless any such murder is not only extremely regrettable, but also raises serious issues as to whether it was possible to prevent it. Inquiry committees set up in the wake of such cases have highlighted the following:[41]

- Most of the people who committed these murders were not in close contact with mental health services.
- Multidisciplinary work was not as well coordinated as it should have been; often one group of workers did not inform the other group of significant developments, and did not attempt to secure joint work.
- Relatives were often kept at arms length and not listened to.
- Users stopped taking their medication some time before the murder took place.
- Nearly all of the victims were known to the killer (32 out of 34), as is usually the case in other murders.
- Murders were committed without provocation, and when the person was influenced by paranoid perceptions.

It would therefore seem that sound multiprofessional practice is required in working with people likely to commit violent offences.

None of these reports mention the lack of asylum facilities in the community, the difficulty users experience in even discussing issues concerning their reluctance to take medication, let alone steps that seriously address their complaints about side-effects, the effect of emotional and social isolation, and the sense of despair that most of these people experience for most of the time. These issues need to be tackled if harm to others is going to be reduced further.

The English National Board, which is responsible for training nurses, recommended in 1993 (circular 1993/11/GMB: 'Coping with Violence and Aggression: Prevention and Management') that training colleges should set up courses focusing on response to violent behaviour. As there is no evidence to suggest that such training has been introduced elsewhere in Europe, we are left to wonder whether the change in Britain is cultural-specific or relates to a specific context created by the reduction of public services and benefits to poor people, and/or whether it is about increased aggression by service users and/or workers.

Following legislation in some North American states, the British government has attempted to legislate a community supervision order.[42] Such an order would allow people to be recalled to hospital and forced to take medication if it is known that they have stopped taking it, even if no deterioration in their mental state can be observed. The government has estimated that between 2000 and 4000 people may fall into this category. This initiative has been supported by the Royal College of Psychiatrists, the Royal College of Psychiatrists, the Royal College of Physicians and Sane (Schizophrenia a national emergency). Significantly it has been *rejected* by all other professional organisations, user groups and the main relatives' organisation (the NSF, the National Schizophrenia Fellowship), and was found wanting by a parliamentary committee in 1993. As an interim measure, a register of continued care clients at risk was introduced in April 1994, even though the criteria for putting people on it are not clear. The debate on this issue continues, reflecting the unease and sense of threat felt by continued care clients living in our midst.

As mentioned above, the likelihood of self-harm by continued care clients – especially those suffering from schizophrenia, personality disorder and depression – is realistically much greater than that of harming others, estimated at 10 per cent of all patients in these categories. This is expressed in various forms of self-defeating behaviour, culminating in anorexia, attempted suicide or completed suicide.

The psychological price of self-harm extends far beyond the individual concerned, to relatives, friends and workers. Yet self-harm was perceived as the only way left to women in Ashworth special hospital to their express anger (as quoted above). Others have suggested that it is a way of purifying oneself, of exercising control, of taking revenge, of daring, and of feeling that there is no other solution but to leave this world.[43]

Most of our planned interventions to prevent self-harm seem to be placed at the level of preventing access to the means of self-harm, force-feeding in the case of anorexia, and attempting to improve the person's well-being in more general ways, for example medication against depression, medication to block psychotic symptoms or attempts to interest the person in more enjoyable activities. Counselling and psychotherapy are used, but less often than the other methods.

People who harm themselves suggest that their needs are little different from those of others: to be loved and accepted, to feel and be safe, and the meeting of basic needs such as shelter, work and income. Some of them also propose that they should be allowed to die if they so choose. They see the use of medication as an indication that their difficulties are to do with a distorted view of reality, brought on by mental illness, and therefore as a denial of their existentialist search and suffering.[44]

Early intervention, better coordination among services and more workers in the community have been proposed as measures that could significantly reduce self-harm.[45] Insofar as mental illness is a reflection of inner turmoil, then the *quality* of the contribution of service providers becomes central. Is it going to be good enough to meet what feels like a high level of emotional deprivation, often in tandem with material and social deprivation?

Ways of working with continued care clients in the community

The range of services has expanded considerably in most European countries since 1980 with the introduction of additional community-based services, such as community mental health teams and centres, day care, supported housing, care management, employment projects, and befriending and advocacy schemes.[46] This section focuses on developments in the *content* and *coordination* of intervention methods and services since 1980.

Farkas[47] has outlined the differences in the focus of treatment (mostly through medication), rehabilitation and care management, the three main areas to be looked at below.

Medication

The most prevalent way of working with this group has been through the use of a variety of antipsychotic drugs. These types of medication, developed mainly since the 1950s, have proven to be very effective in arresting the florid symptoms of psychosis ('positive symptoms'), but not in curing or preventing withdrawal from ordinary living, in terms of energy, interest, social and personal functioning, and a sense of well-being.

Medication has been most effective in treating depression and least effective in treating schizophrenia (and personality disorder, which is not categorised as a psychotic disorder).[48] Medication is quick and simple to administer in comparison with psychological and social interventions; hence its great attraction. According to researchers in this field we are coming closer to understanding how such drugs work and why they work by locating their cellular receptors, identifying dopamine and serotonin receptors and their chemical interactions.[49]

A booklet on the psychopharmacology of schizophrenia, published at the end of 1993 by the British Royal College of Psychiatrists summarises up-to-date US and Canadian research. It begins with the following statement: 'Despite the increase in our knowledge of the mechanisms of action of existing antipsychotic drugs, the discovery of new, more effective antipsychotic drugs has not yet been derived from our theoretical understanding of those mechanisms. The recent rediscovery of clozapine is no exception'.[50] Siris,[51] writing in the same publication and clearly sharing the belief in the positive usefulness of antipsychotic drugs, lists the following side effects while examining the issue of adjunctive medication in the treatment of schizophrenia:

- Extrapyramidal side effects (for example stiffness of the small muscles of the face and/or larynx, resulting in a fixed, vacuous expression and/or a monotonous voice).
- Tardive dyskinesia (involuntary muscle movements of the limbs).
- Poor psychosocial adjustment.
- Dystonic reactions and Parkinsonian stiffness and tremor.
- Subtle effects of akinesia (reduction in normal spontaneity)
- Side effects from anti-Parkinsonian drugs: dry mouth, blurred vision, constipation, memory gaps, reduced perception of the passage of time, greater prevalence of symptoms of tardive dyskinesia.
- Side-effects of antidepressants: orthostatic hypotension, peripheral anticholinergic effects, exacerbation of cardiac conduction defects.

Siris' conclusion is that all of this should be taken into account when deciding which adjunctive medication to offer in addition to the antipsychotic drugs themselves. He also indicates that there is likely to be a depressive base underlying schizophrenia, which should be treated with antidepressants. At no point does Siris consider the possibility that this carefully selected cocktail of drugs serves to mask people's problems.

The conclusion that others (some psychiatrists, such as Breggin, and many users of antipsychotic and adjunctive medication)[52] have come to is more radical. For them the harm of the new (and old) drugs is greater than their benefit, and some of it is irreversible (such as tardive dyskinesia, which reflects a small degree of brain damage). Less radical views have been reflected by other psychiatrists concerning the *overuse* of drugs, and their *abuse* not in terms of quantity alone but in the senseless use of multidrugs. It has been further suggested that this can be improved by more focused training of psychiatrists and GPs.[53]

However none of the critiques coming from within psychiatry seem to have taken on board the justified wish of users not only for fuller information about the effects of drugs, but of a gradual withdrawal programme. A small number of such programmes do exist, where a counsellor and the user work together with a psychiatrist, often as part of a group focusing on the effects of major tranquillisers, in a similar format to that used by groups working on withdrawal from minor tranquillisers.[54] The rarity of such work in relation to major tranquillisers reflects not only the fear of relapse by the professionals involved, but also their lack of belief that people can gradually reduce the level of medication and ultimately stop its use. It also reflects the fact that users' complaints about the effects of medication are not taken seriously enough at the non-research level, and instead they are accused of 'non-compliance'.

Psychotherapy and counselling

It is assumed here that there is a place for psychotherapeutic intervention with continued care clients, which has to be tailored to individual needs, wishes and abilities. Some of the innovations in this area are described in Chapter 6, which looks at professionals.

Recent critiques on psychotherapy, especially psychoanalytic psychotherapy, have portrayed it as an ineffective, brainwashing exercise, at times carried out by people who behave in unethical ways, and as particularly damaging for people suffering from serious mental illness.[55] Nonetheless more and more people are going into therapy in all European countries, usually paying for it themselves. Most of the spokepersons of users' groups in Europe are people who have been categorised as continued care clients who have either managed to withdraw from the use of medication or to reduce its use in direct correlation with the amount of time spent in psychotherapy. They are active and highly intelligent people who, according to their own admission, would not have been able to do what they do without the support received through psychotherapy or counselling.

The wide variety of psychotherapy and counselling techniques, including family therapy, could potentially allow the matching of people to therapies, and not only be a source of confusion. Considerable development has taken place in the last fifteen years in cognitive-behavioural therapy, family therapy focused on adults, psychodynamic psychotherapy, and combinations of these strands.[56] Psychoanalytic therapy with survivors of sexual abuse and people suffering from learning difficulties or personality disorders also offers new possibilities of working with people after a psychotic breakdown.[57]

It is understandable that the investment in time and professional expertise required by this type of intervention is off-putting for politicians. In addition the pain experienced, the need to unlearn, side by side with new learning, may be off-putting for the person and his/her family. Therefore early intervention is the best and quickest option for those who believe in the usefulness of psychotherapy and counselling. Much more up-front, jargon-free information should be made available, and both the research and the ethical base should be closely scrutinised.

Traditional forms of psychotherapy and counselling are unlikely to work well for continued care clients, but there is a positive role to be played by therapists who take on board not only the individualised needs of the user, but also the implications of being a continued care client.

Assertive out-reach programmes

Most of these rehabilitation programmes originated as a result of an acceptance of the limitations of the usefulness of antipsychotic medication and a lack of belief in the efficacy of psychotherapeutic approaches. The programmes were developed by professionals who accepted the importance of the social aspects of the existence of continued care clients as a precondition to their psychological well-being and reintegration to the community.

Such programmes were developed mainly in the United States and Australia, and have been adopted in Britain, Denmark, France, Germany, Italy and the Netherlands by workers who intuitively accept social role valorisation principles. The programmes are based on the assumption that continued care clients require both *assertive* and *continuous* support. Accessibility and flexibility are the hallmarks of the approach. The type of support provided ranges from shopping to medication, sorting out benefits and money matters, home visits, and going on holiday together, according to individual needs. Some of the US programmes have been evaluated over a long time to reveal that they are more effective than other rehabilitation programmes in preventing relapses and hospital admissions.[58] While such programmes require programmes considerable staff input and can be very emotionally demanding on the part of the staff, workers can come from a variety of backgrounds and do not need to be highly qualified (or paid) professionals, as the post-assessment skills needed for this type of work are the ability to be supportive and persistent, rather than being trained in specific intervention techniques. Users have at times found the programmes too intrusive and controlling.

In Europe, attempts to imitate the US models without adaptation have not been very successful.[59]

Ways of working with relatives

The development in *psychoeducative* programmes, exemplified by 'expressed emotions' (outlined in Chapter 2), presents us with an additional and promising way of reaching individuals and their families. Psychoeducative approaches have the advantage of not only providing people with an extended repertoire of coping strategies, but also of fostering less dependency, giving people permission not to experience too much pain (by stirring away from the emotional level), and especially enabling them.

The reported effectiveness of such programmes is high.[60] Interestingly, all these programmes hold a common belief in the biological origin of mental illness. Consequently relatives are discouraged from looking at other perspectives. In principle, psychoeducative programming can be applied within non-biological frameworks too.

Relatives may also benefit from counselling and family therapy. This would depend on the specific approach employed and the sensitivity of the therapist or counsellor in balancing the needs of the relatives as individuals with the needs of the clients. Research on relatives' views of family therapy that focuses on their young children has highlighted their ambivalence and sense of power inequality.[61]

Support groups, with and without professional involvement, have been welcomed by the relatives who participate in them for providing a mixture of emotional and social support with information. Relatives have to be ready to declare themselves as such when joining such a group, and may not find it easy to do so as this confirms the stigma attached to being a relative of a sufferer.

Relatives often complain of being disregarded by professionals, taken for granted and/or blamed for the mental illness of their family member, especially if they are parents. This issue will be looked at further in Chapter 6.

Care coordination

Care coordination has been with us for a long time as part of an efficient service provision. However it has been boosted by programmes of case-care management developed initially in the United States,[62] in part due to the belief that they are more cost effective. It is now also used in The Netherlands and Italy, having been introduced by American psychiatrists.[63] Care management has become prominent as a way of overcoming the past neglect of continued care clients, the lack of coordination and collaboration among different services and professional disciplines, the lack of sufficient involvement by users and relatives, and the insufficient use of non-statutory and informal services.

The approach begins with a renewed focus on identifying and assessing *needs*. The operationalised definition of need according to mainstream psychiatry is:[64] (a) performance in a given area of functioning is falling significantly beyond a specified level (that is, a deficit is present); and (b) a potentially effective intervention must exist to meet the need (that is, the deficit must be potentially remediable). Care management programmes that focus on *strengths and wants* use a non-jargonised ordinary definition of need, as something necessary for living at an acceptable standard, which is currently missing.[65] The difference in approach is important here, because it encapsulates the following differences:

- Is the deficit located in the client's performance, or in conditions that promote/block his/her performance?
- Is need defined only normatively (that is by society, by professionals as representatives of society), or also by the client?
- Are wishes – which go beyond normative deficits – to be recognised as important aspects of people's lives or not?
- Do we want to enable people to achieve their potential, or only to ensure that they function at the minimum socially acceptable level.

Figure 4.1 is a diagrammatic example of the 'problem-focused' approach to care management, which incorporates needs, strengths and the user's personal control in care management.

Within the strength model *wishes* have been utilised as a motivating factor, as a goal to work towards together, as a way of telling the client that his/her *dreams* are important. Even if not always achievable, some elements of their ambitions are worthwhile working towards. Thus wishes – and the work aimed at achieving them – have been used as a tool to empower and enable.

Once the needs have been identified and assessed, the care management process turns to the planning of a care package. The more flexible, individualised and all-involving such a planning exercise is, the better. Those involved should include the user and her/his relatives or friends, the professionals who contributed to the various assessment components, and the care manager. All those involved, but especially the care manager, need to have a good knowledge of local formal and informal services, as well as their costs, and have a good enough information system to enable him/her to learn about faraway services, if

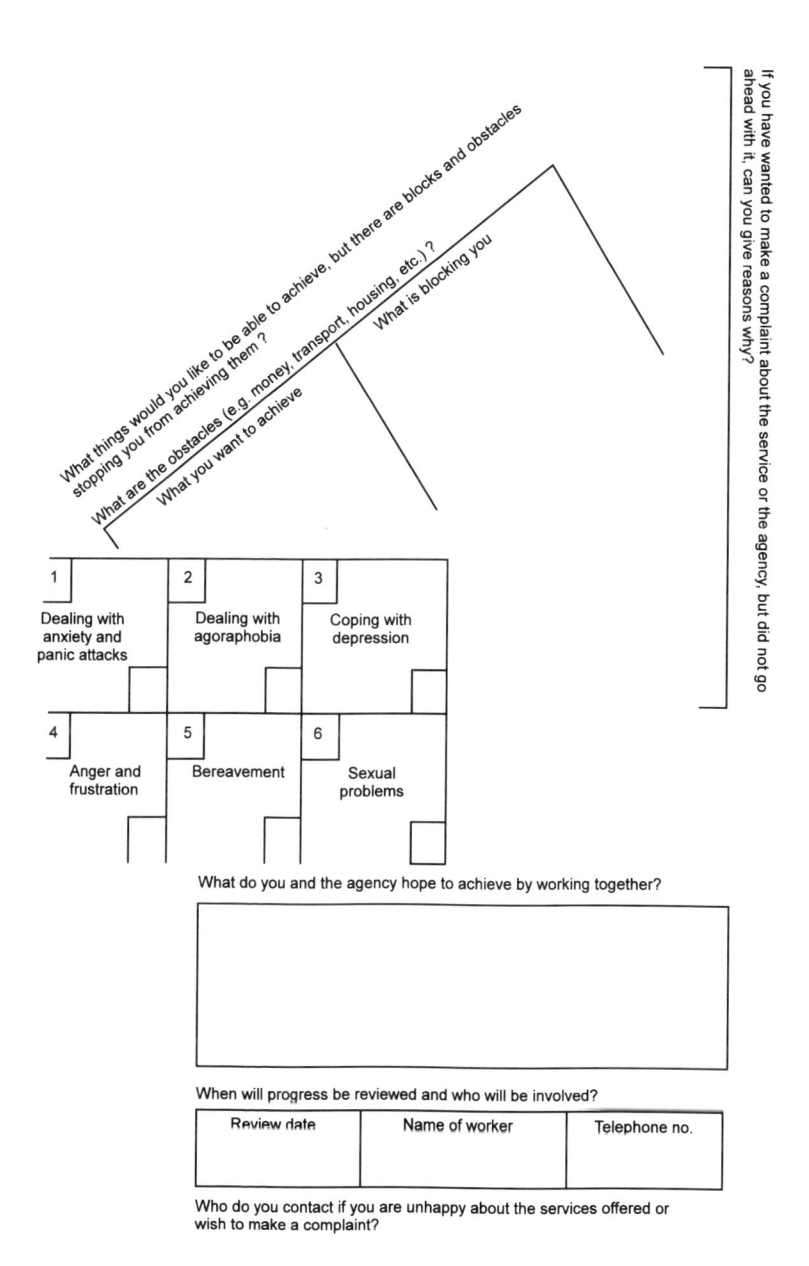

What things would you like to be able to achieve, but there are blocks and obstacles stopping you from achieving them?

What are the obstacles (e.g. money, transport, housing, etc.)?

What you want to achieve

What is blocking you

If you have wanted to make a complaint about the service or the agency, but did not go ahead with it, can you give reasons why?

1 Dealing with anxiety and panic attacks	2 Dealing with agoraphobia	3 Coping with depression
4 Anger and frustration	5 Bereavement	6 Sexual problems

What do you and the agency hope to achieve by working together?

When will progress be reviewed and who will be involved?

Review date	Name of worker	Telephone no.

Who do you contact if you are unhappy about the services offered or wish to make a complaint?

Figure 4.1 Involving service users in their own care management assessment

needed. The agreed package, and the ways of achieving it, can then be implemented.

Care management thus lends itself to the use a mixed-service-sectors approach, to buying/creating/providing individualised services instead of fitting people into existing services, to value information and consultation.

Care management models[66] differ not only in their definition of need and whether or not they focus on wishes and strengths. They also differ in the degree of involvement of users and relatives in the process of care management, the depth of focus on enhancing autonomy through the care package, the length to which the care manager will go to obtain sufficiently good information and services, the involvement of the care manager in service provision, the inbuilt mechanisms of quality assurance, or review and redress, and the degree to which the whole process is determined by cost calculations.

Brokerage[67] is a form of care management in which the client employs an independent person to coordinate the implementation of the care package, following agreement on the package itself with the funding authority. It is similar to the service provided by an advocate, but where the advocate's duty stops at representing the client to others, the broker is there to ensure that things happen, and that the services provide what the client wants. Having a broker also significantly redresses the power imbalance between users and services.

Relatives' own initiatives

The North American relatives organisation, NAMI, has provided a powerful example for European relatives of sufferers.[68] In one specific case that I came across they had adopted a group of relatives in Kiev and offered the group modest financial support, besides advice and moral support. Within two years the group in Kiev – consisting mainly of mothers of young adults suffering from schizophrenia – had:

- Set up monthly support and information meetings.
- Provided legal advice to those wishing to act as guardians for people discharged into the community (to date the only

means of being discharged after compulsory admission is through guardianship);
- Put pressure on the government to provide free medication.
- Entered into a dialogue with hospital administration and secured the right to inspect the physical conditions of the hospital.
- Organised a sheltered workshop facility outside the hospital for young service users, which is producing jewellery.
- Translated the NAMI newsletters into Ukrainian.

Yet the leaders of the group are finding it an uphill struggle to liaise between the members and the authorities. The anger and bitterness among the members – pent up for so many years – has resulted in considerable aggression, at times aimed at the leaders.

British relatives have developed one large organisation (the National Schizophrenia Fellowship, NSF) with 6000 members, as well as many small, unaffiliated groups. Apart from supporting each other, some local groups have branched out into developing group homes and day-care and workshop facilities.[69] The NSF also acts as a pressure group. This includes collating and distributing information, carrying out surveys, finding out what the membership wants, and representing their views to politicians, the media and professionals. The NSF has usually taken the pro-traditional psychiatry line, including the usefulness of rehabilitation.

The Netherlands too has a tradition of relatives' organisations, particularly in the area of learning difficulties. In relation to mental health it seems to be more of a mutual-support and protest movement than a service provider and innovator.[70]

Some similar and some different developments took place in Italy during the 1980s. Writing about the development of a relatives' group in Imola, Soglia,[71] describes their sense of indignation at the conditions in the local psychiatric hospital as providing the impetus for the group's establishment in 1984. As in Kiev, the group consists of women only – mothers and sisters. Initially its aims were to offer emotional and social support and information, but the group is now a service provider and runs residential facilities that broadly follow the social role valorisation approach. However, unlike Britain, Italy has three relatives' organisations and these disagree with each other on the subject of deinstitutionalisation. Their power to exert political pressure is weaker than that enjoyed by the British organisation. This is not only because the three organisations have different objectives, but also because of the less sophisticated ways in which the Italian organisations operate.

Relatives are to be found among the activists of most pressure groups in mental health throughout Europe, even when the specific organisation within which they operate is not a relatives' group *per se*.

Relatives' organisations have moved into service provision in part to fill a vacuum, but mainly due to the introduction of the mixed welfare economy, described in Chapter 1. The issue of whether relatives' organisations should be service providers – as distinct from their mutual support and policy pressure functions – is intriguing. On the one hand it is assumed that because of their experiences they have a better understanding of what users – and their relatives – need. On the other hand users and workers have argued that relatives' understanding is coloured to such an extent that they are unlikely to be able to provide users with what they need and want. But the main underlying issue is that service provision is likely to lead to a new type of dependency on the authorities, which usually fund both the services and the organisations criticised by relatives when in their policy pressure and campaigning mode. Will relatives' groups have to give up campaigning, or be more true to their original mission by giving up service provision?

Similar issues face service users when they move into service provision, and this will be discussed next.

Continued care clients' own initiatives

Users of mental health services have attempted to organise their own networks informally and formally since the nineteenth century. The Finnish Mental Health Association, which began as a users' group, has been in operation since 1897. It now provides:

- training projects, including a three-year course on family therapy;
- rehabilitation training for both users and relatives;
- networking users into existing groups;

- housing projects (together with the Central league for Mental health, a user-only organisation);
- counselling and information;
- a crisis service (SOS Service, focusing on suicide prevention in Helsinki and Lahti).

The Finish organisation exemplifies the pre-1980s organisations, where the aim was to create alliances with interested others, such as relatives and professionals, rather than to keep it as a user-only group.

User-only organisations are more typical of post-1980 developments across Europe, following a greater focus on the rights of minorities, citizenship and antimarginalisation attempts (outlined in Chapter 2). This direction has been in part modelled on the North American user movement, which has demonstrated its ability not only to create a user network, but also to establish user-managed services and representation of users in national and local fora.[72]

The second main influence on the European movement has come from the Netherlands, where two national advocacy organisations have been in existence since the early 1970s.[73] The Client Union and the National Foundation of Patients and Residents Council are user-managed, and provide individual advocacy by advocates who have been/still are service users themselves, as well as leadership in setting up user for a such as patients' councils in hospital wards. The Dutch model has become the prototype for most of the British advocacy schemes. Enabling hospitalised patients to begin to communicate with each other informally on issues of common concern, and to develop the ability to run a meeting and represent themselves to the management, are indeed important achievements and demonstrate that even in the midst of a personal crisis people can – and want to – share, support and contribute towards the improvement of services.

Representing users' interests and views on national planning committees is another achievement of the Dutch movement. Yet a growing number of its founder members have expressed their disappointment with the inability of the movement to bring about the more fundamental changes in the Dutch mental health system that they hoped it would lead to, and acknowledge their relative lack of power in comparison with the power wielded by professionals and politicians.[74] These desired changes were/are about demedicalising the system, following a society-wide attitudinal shift towards greater tolerance of the differences represented by people suffering from mental distress.

While expressing their disappointment, to date an analysis of this state of affairs is lacking. Such an analysis is likely to indicate the role of co-optation by the establishment as a means of keeping users quiet, but also the absence of systematic work on alternative visions and systematic investment in these alternatives, in alliance with professionals and politicians who are ready to move in this direction. Thorny issues such as how to understand and handle risk of harm to others and self-harm would also need to be addressed in such an analysis.

Users' own organisations now exist throughout Europe. A useful summary was published by the European User Network in 1992, listing such organisations in thirteen countries, varying in size from 45 members in a Polish group to 10 000 in a Swedish organisation. A more recent publication by the European Regional Council illustrates the growth of such initiatives.[75] The focus in this section is on the services that such groups provide.

All groups offer *mutual support* and *consciousness-raising*, which ease some of the suffering and the experience of being stigmatised, as well as informing people of the range of coping strategies available. Thus the groups play a crucial role in rebuilding threatened identities (a concept discussed in Chapter 2). Some groups offer a drop-in facility, where people can meet in a relaxed environment and decide on the activities they wish to engage in, as well as providing sessional services, often focussing on *information* and *advice*.

The Prato self-help group, initiated by a psychiatrist influenced by the British user movement, has its own management committee, runs a number of social activities (including a theatre group, which performs to the general public), and is actively involved in setting up Italy's national mental health association.[76] It is supported by the health authority, a Catholic, left-wing cultural association, and a social care cooperative – a mixture that indicates the number of hitherto untapped resources in the different European communities.

In a recent meeting of the management committee of Prato I met S., the secretary, a young and vivacious woman; G., a middle-aged woman who spoke about the opportunities the group offered her to write and recite poetry; R, a young man who was unable to sit through the meeting and disrupted the discussion by joking, moving around, leaving the room and coming back several times (a behaviour that was tolerated in a relaxed manner by the rest of the group); A., a worker of the cultural association; P., a psychiatrist; and L, a nurse who is initiating a new self-help group in another part of the town.

The meeting took place in the upstairs room of a local coffee bar; soft drinks were available. The people at the bar below knew of the group's formal name and seemed to treat it as any other local group. Most of the discussion was about the activities planned for the forthcoming mental health day on 10 October, a consciousness-raising event intended to involve the local community, not just service users. The focus was on activities that would attract ordinary people, the media and local politicians. An interesting undercurrent was about who would represent the group, reflecting an internal struggle between S., the secretary, and A., the support worker. A lot of gentle bantering took place.

This group typifies an organisation in the making, where the initiative has come from non-users, as has been the case in most countries at the initial stage of establishing a user movement. The balance of power is fragile, and the users will need to have much more experience of running a group before they will be able to take full control. Will such control be given to them by the professionals involved, all of whom seem to be dedicated to the group and have invested in it beyond the call of duty?

Survivors Speak Out (SSO)[77] is a national British user movement, in which individual service users are full members with voting rights and others can be allies. The idea was first proposed by a psychologist, who is also a relative of a person suffering from mental illness. The founder members were at the time (the mid 1980s) participants in the British Network for Alternatives to Psychiatry (a branch of a European network initiated by the Italian psychiatric reform group), consisting of both professionals and users. In SSO committee membership is open to users only.

The organisation provides a newsletter and an information service, and is involved in preparing a crisis card system, providing training and representing its members' views to professionals, politicians and the media. It has an active poetry group, which both publishes poetry and holds readings. SSO is sponsored by two public grant-making national organisations in this field, but many of its activities are provided by members on a voluntary basis. From time to time members disappear or reappear – those in the know are aware that another mental distress crisis is being experienced, at times ending in hospitalisation.

Thus a range of services is offered by continued care clients to other continued care clients, and/or by exservice users. This reflects the strength that people assumed to be disabled have, and the largely untapped potential still to be brought to the fore.

In a recent publication Lindow[78] provided useful guidelines on self-help alternatives to mental health services. The booklet illustrates both the necessary conditions for a successful self-help venture, and the wide scope that such schemes have. Most of the examples are taken from the United States; a minority from Britain, Canada and New Zealand. As the Dutch, Finish and Italian examples discussed above highlight, self-help alternatives are not limited to the Anglo-Saxon culture. Yet the question of adapting self-help to local cultural forms needs to be addressed, rather than assuming that Europe has to follow Anglo-Saxon patterns.

However the issue of whether the entire mental health service system should – or could – be provided by service users and exusers remains open. This is particularly true of services that require a constant and long-term presence. At the same time, users' perceptions about services have proven most valuable in improving services and approaches.

A related and interesting issue is what happens to the identity of users who become workers in user-run services. Do the two identities (user and worker) merge, coexist or conflict? Does one take over the other periodically, or for good? What is it like to be a 'professional user'? In her frank and descriptive article. Viv Lindow questions whether she is a 'Survivor, Activist or Witch',[79] and looks at the uncomfortable coexistence of her different roles and identities, and the personal cost of putting to good use her experience of the psychiatric system. The differences between 'abolitionists' (of the medical approach to mental illness) and 'reformists' (that is, those content to continue to change the psychiatric system from within), have also been described by Van Hoorn,[80] and are often about emphasis and style rather than substance. Both groups share the wish to create an alternative service structure to the one that predominates in

Europe at present. Yet the issue of co-optation is particularly alive in terms of service funding and control. The attitude towards the medical model may also oscillate over time, at times reflecting levels of individual suffering.

Despite the notable achievements to date of the various European user groups, the movement as a whole is a long way away from being able to provide a full alternative service or change social attitudes to the point of radically restructuring European mental health services. As suggested in connection with the impact of the feminist movement on working with women service users, there is considerable scope for the further development of user-run services, provided the limitations of such a development are taken on board.

Summary

Our knowledge of continued care clients, our attitudes towards them and their relatives, the ways of working with and for them, as well as their own contribution, have changed considerably since 1980. Europe has been able to rediscover them as people, and consequently to allow them to rediscover themselves and influence our perception of them.

With the rediscovery of continued care clients came the rediscovery of their relatives, the stresses they face, their wishes, strengths and weakness. This dual discovery has heightened the profile of continued care clients in our societies, albeit often in conflicting forms.

While most of this process has provided more positive results than those obtained in the past when working with this client group, we are also facing the possibility of the reintroduction of greater coercive control and the criminalisation of a minority within this heterogeneous group.

5
Innovations in Housing and Employment

Introduction

The closure of psychiatric hospitals has forced our attention to housing as never before, as planners have become convinced that the success or failure of such closures will depend on finding appropriate housing solutions. While service users have been arguing that employment is as essential as housing for an ordinary life in the community, planners have hardly taken on board the creation of work opportunities.

Housing: needs and wishes

Our awareness of housing issues for people suffering from mental illness has become more acute not only due to hospital closure, but especially as homelessness became more visible on European streets during the 1980s and 1990s. Housing for people suffering from the effects of long-term mental illness has always been a distressing issue as it encapsulates:

- the breakdown of previous living arrangements;
- often the need to move away from one's family after the internal relationships have deteriorated to the point where living together cannot be tolerated;
- while hospitalised, being evicted for rent arrears;
- finding oneself without a roof, on someone else's sofa or in a night shelter;
- being without a job and at times without any state support.

Most of us take for granted the availability of a place to live that is also our home. Having a home meets our need for safety, privacy, health and an individualised life-style, as well as providing a place to return to, stability, shelter and a place where one can invite others. Having a home is also a necessary condition for a sustained recovery from a mental distress crisis, as well as being a preventive measure. In order to obtain a job, people are required to have a permanent address.

Most of us would find it difficult, if not impossible, to imagine what it is like not to have a home at any point in our lives. This makes our encounters with homeless people uncomfortable and complex, as we may see the situation as too horrendous to empathise with, feel personally guilty, or be unable to understand and communicate with homeless people.

We also take it for granted that people will be ready to accept *any* housing solution rather than be without a home, and we are surprised when this proves not to be the case. We may then conclude that 'they' do not wish to have a home, that they are ungrateful. We may, wash our hands of them and punish them when their visibility is too upsetting for us to witness. Research on homeless people reveals that nearly all of them would like to have a home, but are not necessarily ready to accept the constraints and responsibilities that having a home entails.[1]

Between 30 per cent and 50 per cent of all homeless people are assumed to suffer from serious mental illness, though this is based on rough estimates rather than research.[2] In remand centres the figure is likely to be higher. For example 75 per cent of people remanded in Brixton Prison (South London) in 1993 were found to suffer from both homelessness and mental illness,[3] illustrating how difficult it is to disentangle the debate on what comes first, homelessness or mental illness. Contrary to the claims made by some psychiatrists and relatives' pressure groups, virtually no long-stay patients become homeless.[4]

In a recent review article, Scott[5] suggested that we need to be aware of the existence of three subgroups of people who are both homeless and suffer from mental illness so that their needs may be recognised and services planned accordingly:

- people with a history of hospitalisation who become homeless some time after their discharge from hospital;
- younger people who avoid psychiatric intervention and whose mental illness 'may have contributed to social drift' (ibid., p. 321);
- people who became mentally ill due to homelessness, or the

personal/social problem that led them to become homeless in the first place.

Current changes in housing schemes ownership

A considerable growth in the number of housing schemes for people with mental distress took place in the 1980s throughout Europe, in response to hospital closures and to the preference for maintaining people in the community. As a result of the move towards mixed welfare sectors (outlined in Chapter 1), most of the new schemes and a large proportion of the older ones have become privately owned. Within this emerging private sector the majority of the schemes are owned by not-for-profit organisations and are largely paid for by social security funding. Unlike in the United States, the expected takeover by large for-profit corporations has not happened, perhaps due to the less lucrative European market.

This change also has implications for the mechanisms that are necessary for *quality assurance*. Adequate inspection arrangements have to be put in place by the funding organisation or a watchdog agency – inspection not only of physical living conditions, but also of how residents are treated and the opportunities provided for their integration to the community. These last two dimensions are more difficult to assess and require more than a fleeting visit.

The ownership of housing schemes by not-for-profit organisations (yet another example of the quasi-market) has additional and important implications for the character of the not-for-profit voluntary sector. By becoming a *provider* agency, which depends on statutory services for the renewal of its contract, such an agency is likely to be less active in its *campaigning activities* and less active in involving lay, unpaid people in its overall activities, and more likely to become a business-orientated organisation.

Housing solutions

Hospital placements

Hospital hostels, or hospital 'wards in the community',[6] have been experimented with since the early 1980s. These are intended as long-term – though not necessarily permanent – solutions for people who have been hospitalised in conjunction with offences and/or challenging behaviour. For those judged to be either unable to live in the community or too risky to others and themselves, hospital hostels aim to provide a more ordinary environment, with greater privacy, freedom and responsibility for self-care and communal living. While most hostels provide an environment that is more akin to a hospital than an ordinary living environment, in one such recently established scheme[7] residents are involved in staff selection as well as in choosing to move to the hostel in the first place.

In Trieste and Arezzo the older and more physically and psychologically dependent expatients live in group homes on the premises of the old hospitals.[8] A number of other projects unrelated to mental health services are also taking place, such as the Faculty of Humanities of the University of Trieste and a secondary school for vocational training in Arezzo, beside facilities that are part of the new structure of mental health services, such as community mental health centres, work cooperatives, and research and education centres. The residents of these sheltered flats have their own keys, and in line with the general policy on group homes care staff are not available during the night. Thus the homes are run like any other group home for elderly people, and not like a variation of a hospital ward. Given that the two ex-hospitals are located in residential areas the residents are not too isolated from the ordinary life of the towns.

Family placements

Family placements are one of the oldest solutions to housing problems, though one that has hardly been evaluated. Gheel in Flemish Belgium is renowned for its system of foster families for adults formerly hospitalised in the local psychiatric institution, many of whom have learning difficulties. This system has been in operation since the eighteenth century. Those fostered live and work with the foster family. In many cases they look after their elderly foster parents after the natural children have left the town. No antagonistic reactions have been reported among the residents of the city, but anthropological research by Roosnes[9] has highlighted the fact that they are kept at arms' length socially (for example they are not members of the local church), that they are made fun of in the local drinking place, and that they can be recalled to the hospital without a formal procedure of reinvestigation.

Jodelet[10] has studied a similar example in France over a period of four years. Two small French towns, Dur-sur-Arun and Ainey-le-Chateau, have had a family colony since 1892 and 1900 respectively. Jodelet's research focused on Ainey-le-Chateau, situated only four hours from Paris. During the 1980s 1195 people lived as lodgers with 493 families. Lodgers were selected by psychiatrists from among those who did not exhibit behavioural problems. Outpatient appointments and domiciliary visits were offered. The initial fear expressed in 1900 soon subsided, with comments such as 'For madmen they are very quiet', 'you would think they were quite middle class', and 'if you did not know you would never guess' being made as early as 1901.[11]

Sixty per cent of the 1195 lodgers lived in small, relatively poor flats and houses, 31 per cent in medium-sized farms and 8 per cent in large farm estates. A further distinction was made as to the space within the household occupied by the lodger–patient, some of whom were separated from the family by being put into outhouses or sheds while others had a room in the family home. These arrangement had implications for the availability of running water and heating, as well as for the degree of inclusion in or exclusion from the family and its activities, including unpaid work.

The host families were paid the cost of housing and full board, so it is not surprising that this arrangement appealed more to poorer families or individuals. Forty-one per cent of heads of families at the time of Jodelet's research were unemployed.[12] The family colony has become the major industry of the town, in the same way that psychiatric hospitals are the main industry in places such as Leros in Greece and in rural Ireland. This economic dependency creates its own tension and adds to the ambivalence surrounding such placements.

Most of Jodelet's fascinating study focuses on the way the lodgers were treated by the inhabitants of Ainey-le-Chateau, and the significance of this on views and attitudes towards madness and people defined as mad. Despite – or because of – their close proximity and shared activities, the locals demonstrated considerable apprehension and suspicion towards the lodgers, most of which was not based on any actual behaviour by the latter. The lodgers were perceived as not fully human, even if distinctions were made between those who were more with it, and those who were not. Fear of their sexuality, rather than possible aggression, seemed to be lurking. There were known instances of sexual relationships between lodgers and non- lodgers, and of children being born of these relationships.

A number of physical and imaginary barriers seemed to have been erected by the locals to distance themselves from the lodgers. Jodelet suggests that the aim of the barriers and the distance was to ensure that the ordinary inhabitants would not be viewed by others or by themselves as tainted by their madness as a result of residing in such close proximity.

Those who became too close to lodgers had to pay a price. While children by lodgers were tolerated, though gossiped about, marriage to them was perceived as taboo, and those few who did marry lodgers went to live elsewhere with them: '. . . and then there was Mademoiselle . . . who had one staying with her who was her lover for twenty years. She's left now, lives with him somewhere near Vichy. She's married'.[13]

The less-than-human perception is demonstrated in the following quotation:

> 'Have you heard what happened today?'
> 'No.'
> 'There were two Swiss women who were out of luck. They ran over a patient. It was because of the tobacco. He must have been feeling unwell. There are some who say it's like suicide. I think he was unwell. Just before he'd said to the other bloke, "I don't feel well". The doctor came. At the Colony they come straightaway in cases like that. Once the report has been made, there's nothing else to do. They went on their way, the poor women'.[14]

Although not living in mini-institutions, the lodgers remained institutionalised by virtue of their legal status as patients, and by being placed in an arrangement in which they were treated as though they were constantly on the verge of a breakdown.

It is regrettable that this most interesting study does not include the views and feelings of the lodgers. Although conducted in the 1980s, it is as if the researcher – a distinguished social psychologist in Paris – did not consider the need to incorporate the users' own perspectives as an integral part of her work. What did it feel like to be the recipient of all this ambiguity, fear and distancing? What was its impact on people who had already gone through a major crisis, had been hospitalised and moved/removed from their initial homes only to become the subject of such an approach by people with whom they lived and were dependent upon? These are just some of the questions awaiting further anthropological study. Jodelet's social representation approach treats the patient–lodgers as objects of study rather than participants in a human drama.

Most other family placements are arranged on an individual basis, rather than on the large scale available in Gheel and Ainey-le-Chateau, and are supported by social workers rather than a psychiatric service. Family placements can meet a number of needs, such as safety, health, shelter, a place to return to and stability. Despite enabling the patient–lodgers to take part in ordinary living, such placements tend to fall short of enabling them to become part of an ordinary primary grouping or to encourage them to engage in inside or outside ordinary activities. Despite the fact that family homes are treated as a private space, lodgers do not seem to have the right to privacy or the right to invite guests to the home. While there are kind landladies and lodgers who benefit from such kindness, distancing and indifference are also likely to prevail.

Group homes

Such homes have been established since the 1960s, when the number of people leaving psychiatric hospitals and the rate of discharge began to increase, and the length of stay began to decrease. Group homes require considerable planning, capital investment and revenue, as well as preparing the residents-to-be, selecting staff and maintaining the homes.

In an attempt to prevent reinstitutionalisation in the community, most group homes have no more than eight residents. However it would seem that the *regime* of the homes and the perceptions of the staff are more crucial than the actual number of residents.[15] In most homes residents are expected to carry out some components of everyday maintenance and are responsible for looking after their own rooms. They are also expected to respect rules governing shared areas and to exhibit cordial behaviour towards neighbours. There are many variations pertaining to rules on everyday living, for example with respect to smoking, residents having their own key, defending privacy by preventing non-invited people from entering individual rooms, having guests and friends to stay, whether sexual activity is formally prohibited or not, the degree of tolerance of psychiatric symptoms and refusal to take medication, control over money, the choice of menu, clothing, furniture and outdoor activities, the choice of whether or not to attend day activities, and the availability of house meetings. Group homes also differ in whether or not there are around-the-clock staff, in the degree of encouragement given to residents to organise activities on their own, and in the effort put into moving residents on to more independent living schemes and/or finding employment opportunities. Most homes do not allow the use of drugs or alcohol, beyond social drinking.

Some of these decisions are related to the assumed level of residual mental illness and difficulties in coping, while others depend more on the philosophy underlying the housing policy and the degree of commitment to provide an ordinary living environment. To date, few housing schemes have also focused on providing opportunities for a *valued* life.

The *geographical* location of a group home reflects the intentions of the planners. The several group homes available in Trieste outside the grounds of the closed hospital have a younger group of residents (although there are a number of residents aged 55 and over), less staff cover and more autonomy for the residents. The homes are undistinguishable from other houses in the same street. One flat, situated within an ordinary apartment block, is used as a drop-in and social club for the younger group, and is served by volunteers and the young users themselves. It is imaginatively and beautifully furnished by the carpentry work co-operative of the mental health services, and is soundproofed.[16]

In Britain planners, and care staff, assume that group home life should resemble family life as much as possible. Given that most staff members are younger than the ex-long-stay patients who have become residents, the family image is an illusion in which everyone is expected to collude. It is as if planners do not believe that it is possible for a group of people to enjoy communal living without being a family unit.[17] At the same time, group homes have few links with the neighbourhood in which they are located, the residential life-style is regimented and the staff tend to interpret disagreement as a sign of pathology, of which they are afraid.

Clinically diagnosed symptomatology does not increase after leaving hospital. Relatively few readmissions take place. The main gains are improved social performance, improved self-care ability and an overall improvement in the quality of life of residents in comparison with hospital living.[18] This range of findings shows that psychiatric symptomatology is an insufficient predictor of people's ability to lead a supported life in the community, as well as illustrating once more that most of the residents did not need to remain in hospital for the long periods that they had spent there.

Recent research has revealed that the cost of accommodation is continuing to increase and accounts for 75–90 per cent of all spending on this client group. In some instances the cost of accommodation is reported as being higher than the cost of hospital treatment, unlike previous reports.[19] This may be the case for the minority of ex-patients perceived to be at risk to themselves and others in the community, or those exhibiting challenging behaviour. However in all cases hospital treatment did not include the range of activities enjoyed by the participants in the schemes and did not lead to the improvements in self-care and ability to communicate demonstrated by the residents a year after leaving hospital. The figures also illustrate the relatively low investment in non-housing services, which could have reduced the need for 24-hour staff cover in a number of houses, and thus could have led to a reduction in the overall cost of the accommodation component. The cost of housing is central to the debate about the financial viability of closing hospitals and relying on services in the community.

Inflexibility and fear of risk may prevent readiness to reduce staff cover when it becomes unproductive. For example it took one housing association three years(!) to change the status of the house from one that required night staff to one that did not from the time that the residents initiated the request, and after the local police, fire-brigade, health and social services had given their blessing to this change.[20] The wish for change came about two years after the move from the hospital, when the residents had become more confident about being on their own during the night, wanting to use the staff for the purpose of supporting them in outside activities.

Group homes have their crises too. In one group home I recently visited two people committed suicide within two years of leaving hospital, both of them unexpectedly, even though one had attempted suicide before. It is unclear how the other residents felt about these events, as no on-going internal investigation into this issue had taken place. Staff members were badly shaken, though the inquest did not blame them in any way for the suicides. More safety measures were introduced, which meant less responsibility and less privacy for the residents, but greater assurance that suicide would not take place again on the premises. The decision to soft-peddle the issue and not to confront it in a residents' meeting was an understandable strategy, but one that speaks volumes about residents being treated as less than usual tenants.

Most group homes do not have residents from the younger age group, defined as the 'new long stay'. This is partly by design, as the homes are planned for resettled ex-long-stay patients, most of whom tend to be above the age of 50. To introduce younger people, especially those who have not spent as many years in hospital, is tricky. It is likely that their housing needs are best met in stages, rather than by one permanent placement. Yet often the failure of the service is laid at the door of this client group.

A new housing scheme in Nottingham[21] is attempting to take on board the needs and wishes of this younger group, together with the fact that they tend to be more articulate and aware of their rights than the older group. This means that they are likely to be more demanding, less acquiescent and more in need of an income to spend on leisure activities. In fact the younger people involved in the new scheme have expressed a greater need/wish for privacy, and a preference not to live in a group home. The example from Trieste cited above illustrates that it is possible to pay more focused attention to the needs and wishes of this group within the remit of a mental health service.

Core and cluster housing schemes

These schemes aim to provide a greater degree of variety and flexibility in housing options. At the centre of such schemes there is usually a fully staffed facility for people who are deemed to require 24-hour support. This type of facility has a central office and space for communal activities. Either surrounding this or nearby, less staff-supported options are available, such as shared and single flats, facilities for people suffering from physical disabilities as well as mental distress, and at times facilities for people suffering from dementia. It is assumed that moving within the service from one scheme to another is less traumatic for both the resident and the organisation. Furthermore such a scheme enables the staff group to serve more than one facility, and hence it is likely to be more efficient than other schemes. It also offers residents the opportunity to get to know a larger number of people and participate in a greater variety of activities.

At the same time, core and cluster schemes can be seen as reproducing segregation and transinstitutionalisation, as they are likely to be more self-contained and less likely to encourage residents to take make use of outside facilities.

Therapeutic communities

These communities began in the 1940s in Britain, within hospitals as specialised services for soldiers. They also exist inside hospitals in other European countries.[22] In Britain the Richmond Fellowship began to establish such communities outside hospitals from the late 1960s, though the overall number has dwindled considerably since the beginning of the 1980s. This reduction is due to increases in costs at a time of cost cutting, and reservations as to whether the communities – which are more expensive than most other housing solutions – provide a superior service.

Unlike other housing solutions, therapeutic communities also cater for adolescents and younger children suffering from severe mental distress. In Turin a therapeutic community has been established on the third floor of a mental health centre. The setting caters specifically for young people up to the age of 25, who can live there for up to two years. Its proximity to the mental health centre has advantages and disadvantages. For example the residents can use the drop-in cum-cafe on the ground floor of the centre. The stigma attached to having an address identified by others as a mental health centre is one of the drawbacks.

A recent study of one such community in Glasgow Huntly Lodge,[23] indicated that its objectives were the relief of social and psychological difficulties, assisting individuals to find their own identity and a legitimate and valued place within the community. The way towards achieving this complex goal was through the use of responsible client participation in group settings.

At the time of the study (1991) Huntly Lodge had 22 residents, most of them younger than 35, with a history of repeated short admissions. Most had been victims of sexual abuse. Thus Huntly Lodge was one of the relatively few facilities for the new long stay group. The seven staff members provided 24-hour cover. Residents could stay for up to two years, and the cost was covered by the Residential Care Allowance (a social security benefit available to people with a high level of need). The structured daily programme consisted mainly of different group activities, shared house hold chores and weekly individual counselling sessions with a key worker. All this was laid out in a contract signed by both resident and staff.

The evaluation of the scheme focused mainly on the residents' views in comparison with those in a large number of different housing schemes. The areas of symptomatology and quality of life, and the interaction between the two, were investigated. More of the residents of Huntly Lodge suggested that their lives had changed for the better, as well as wishing for a radical change in their lives in the future delete.[24] However the assessment of their psychosocial functioning did not demonstrate such a high degree of change or of their reaching the point of satisfactory functioning.[25] Most of the residents wanted to move to a place of their own.

While such a wide-ranging comparison does not allow conclusive evaluation, it does not appear that Huntly Lodge has led to superior outcomes, but it has been more successful than other schemes in *motivating* residents to change.

Individualised tenancies

This arrangement seems to be service users' preferred housing solution.[26] It is also the preferred way of living for the majority of the general European population. Yet there are numerous instances of people being unable to pay their rent on time and/or look after their flats/houses properly, as well as frequent complaints of loneliness on the part of the users and complaints by neighbours of the users' socially undesirable behaviour. These instances indicate that individualised tenancies are not the best solution for people who are vulnerable in some aspects and who do not have a supportive network around them. It is also an indictment of the over-individualised Western European lifestyle.

To be successful, individualised tenancies require the support of professionals or, preferably, a mixture of lay people and professionals to help with issues such as loneliness, managing budgets and maintaining a home, reflecting once more the underlying need to secure a valued and satisfying personal and social role for these individuals.

For example, Lucy is a community psychiatric nurse in a commercially busy part of inner London. She has been supporting Chris and Jane, both long-term users of mental health services, who live in a flat in a large local housing estate. Many of the flats were bought by the tenants in the relatively recent government push to privatise local authority housing stock. Chris and Jane are usually more active during the night than during the day, at times drinking and quarrelling. Recently their neighbours have complained bitterly of their behaviour and approached the local MP, who in turn approached the local authority and health service. Lucy is worried that Chris and Jane may find themselves even more isolated than they have been up to now, but she also understands the neighbours' concerns. As part of a service innovation project she is planning to establish closer links with the local residents' association and engage in a dialogue about how they would wish to be supported by professionals, but also how they could support Chris and Jane. In addition she is attempting to find some more interesting daytime activities for the couple.

Employment

Unlike housing, employment is not seen as a basic need or a basic citizen's right. This relates to the fact that employment is less about freedom from a threat, as housing is, and more about freedom to fulfil oneself, to enhance one's social position and to contribute to society. Employment is closely linked to individual abilities and motivation, as well as to market competition and availability.

During the last decade we have learned a lot more about the impact of unemployment on ordinary people of all social classes than we have about employment. Research has demonstrated time and again the devastating impact that unemployment, especially long-term unemployment, has on people's aspirations, self-confidence, and physical and mental health.[27] It also negatively affects family relations, and impacts on public expenditure in terms of spiralling unemployment, housing and invalidity benefit costs.

Yet both professionals and lay people continue to deny that unemployment may be acting as a trigger for anxieties that have been repressed more or less successfully for a long time, and that unemployed people and those who share their lives may require counselling, besides material support and help with finding a new job. Janet Mattinson and her colleagues from the Tavistock Institute of Marital Relations have illustrated both the denial and the value of such support in their action research project on families and unemployment, carried out in a London social services department in the mid-1980s.[28] It proved to be really difficult to get referrals from social workers and general practitioners, who kept saying that though their caseloads included unemployed clients, and though many of these clients were married, they did not seem to be experiencing marital problems. Women clients with unemployed partners were not considered spontaneously by their key worker as in need of help with their marital relations, which were likely to have deteriorated as a result of unemployment. However the level and intensity of the misery unearthed by the team in their meetings with couples tells us the exact opposite.

Work not only has a beneficial influence, but like all major structuring facets of our lives it has both a positive and a negative impact on us. To sustain people experiencing difficulties in their jobs is to act in a way that prevents them from having a breakdown in the near future, and prevents them from becoming unemployed. The German Psycho-Social Services (PSS) offers a consistent contact person to the client, and if required the client may also contact the line manager.[29] In addition the service offers courses on work and psychiatric problems. There is little doubt as to the significance of employment in terms of people's self-and social identity and status, as well as their ability to make basic decisions about how to spend their income. Therefore employment – like housing – should be a core component in the rehabilitation of people who suffer from mental illness, if the principles of normalisation and social role valorisation are to be taken seriously. This is patently not the case, as the lack of attention to employment in each successive publication about mental distress demonstrates.[30] We need to understand why this is so.

In a rare study of whether and how inpatients were prepared for employment during their hospitalisation, followed up by an interview three months later when they were living in the outside world, Birch[31] documented the near-absence of such preparation even for people who had been engaged in work before being admitted to hospital. In the three-months post-hospitalisation period, neither work nor the pursual of voluntary service or organised leisure activities were focused upon by the professionals working with these service users.

It would seem that work and employment are not discussed in relation to people suffering from mild forms of mental distress because it is assumed that they will have no difficulty in finding and retaining employment. It is not discussed seriously in the context of severe mental distress because of the assumption that people in this category will be unable to work for a long time, perhaps for ever. It is not discussed with women who are mothers of young children as they are not supposed to have a career anyhow, and it is not discussed with men and women over 50 who are expected to retire ten or fifteen years later. It is not discussed with anyone who is unemployed because we would not wish to upset them as there are so few jobs to go round anyway. This caricatured version of the truth reflects the fact that most professionals in health and social services do not consider employment to be part of their brief.

This inattention by professionals spills over into day activities. Shepherd[32] notes that staff in day centres are reluctant to provide work opportunities for the clients of the centres due to the ambivalence created by the sense of contradiction between 'being sick' and 'being able to work'. The rigid demarcation lines of the implications of the social roles of being ill versus being a worker seem to be at play here.

In contrast service users have put employment as only second to housing on their list of needs to be met,[33] illustrating their awareness of the interaction between being in paid work and being socially valued. Marlieke de Jonge of the Dutch User Movement has succinctly expressed the benefits of work for users:[34]

- It provides a time structure, which gives life a more concrete meaning.
- It widens people's social horizon, including more distanced emotional relationships than those usually experienced within the family.
- It provides an experience of interdependency within a collective framework.
- It enhances status and social identity.
- It makes people active, and forces them to keep fit and take care of themselves so that they are able to work.

I would add that it requires self-discipline, postponement of immediate gratification in many cases, and a well-earned sense of achievement and pride in some instances. The lack of professional attention to work is based on the assumption that most continued care clients are unable to work, and the best they can hope for is to be part of non-work, leisure activities.

Indeed many people in this category are not able to master the skills that most jobs call for – nor can they muster the type of self-discipline that goes with those skills – in the immediate post-hospitalisation period. This is due in part to the effect of medication, and in part to the sharp decline in self-confidence that results from the distressing crisis they have gone through, as well as the effects of the stigma attached to being labelled mentally ill.

However it is argued here that this does not imply that work should not be focused on even at an early stage of hospitalisation. We are all aware of the importance being motivated to return to ordinary life, and especially to employment. By not mentioning the subject the user is indeed receiving the message that those working with him/her believe that work is no longer a realistic option for him/her. Getting back into the habit of looking after oneself and one's environment, and of giving to others are essential components of being a good worker (and a good human being), and furthermore they can be addressed successfully even within the hospital environment. This has been demonstrated in a number of initiatives among therapeutic communities within hospitals, and by the Italian reformers when they began to desegregate the hospitals.[35]

The crucial period for making the first steps towards looking for a job or training is the first few weeks after discharge. At that time people are relieved to have come out of the crisis and are hoping for a full recovery, but are unsure of their future. They may still be too full of medication to be able to do much, and this implies that the dosage may be too strong. This is the time for being befriended, for going to see what types of activity they could join now as a first step towards employment. It would be foolish to propose that most people can walk into a job immediately after discharge, though some could. But they can be encouraged back into a working environment, or to participate in a service where they could provide a positive contribution. Working within a supportive group – such as a cooperative or a social firm – could do the trick.

The Fountain Club was established in the United States, and then in Britain and The Netherlands, with just this in mind.[36] The club offers a high level of enjoyable activities side by side with a high level of user involvement in running the club. It also connects people to educational facilities, and later to jobs. In the club users are encouraged to experiment with a number of activities and then to focus on those activities in which they wish to train. The club also provides a support network when they move into an ordinary work environment.

Clive is a young man of 25 who has been hospitalised a number of times for severe depression and self-harm. At the club he is responsible for the members' newsletter, using his ability to write and his wish to develop it further. Editing the newsletter makes it necessary for him to communicate with others inside and outside the club, something he found difficult in the past. He continues to be shy, and is not sure how he comes across to other people, but he produces a newsletter that others in the club enjoy reading and to which more of them are contributing than was initially the case. He even went with Mark, the club director, to conduct a training session for a group of professionals. This he found scary, but he did it!

Yet such a club is not everyone's cup of tea, and clubs differ according to their directors, other workers, members, the agency and the area in which they operate. A recent survey of users canvassed as to whether they would like to have a club found that they did not; they preferred a real work project, to the amazement of the worker who conducted the survey, who – together with other professionals – was already hooked on the idea of the desirability of a club.[37] The users may be unrealistic in assuming that they can jump the stage that the club provides, but they may be right in assuming that a real work project is a better alternative in that it allows for a more realistic testing of attitudes and abilities, as well as real gains. Thus a lot can be done at the individual level to make employment a realistic objective.

However individual readiness would need to be matched by the availability of suitable jobs. Such availability is known to depend on the general level of unemployment. Yet at any time there is a need for collective action to be taken to secure jobs for people recovering from a mental distress crisis because their vulnerability makes them less able to project the level of abilities and confidence that the world of work takes for granted. Also, collective action can offer more opportunities for jobs that suit users' abilities and wishes, instead of 'safer' but more boring jobs. Zeelen and van Weeghel[38] have proposed a useful framework that incorporates four complementary functions of vocational rehabilitation:

1. Preparation for work: work orientation and training.
2. Transition into work: job searching and finding, trial placements, trainee posts.
3. Assistance in sheltered work projects or social firms: creating such possibilities and supporting those working in existing projects.
4. Support in open employment: outreach care to workers experiencing psychiatric problems; adaptation of the work environment to the needs of this group.

Two structural disincentives need to be addressed to facilitate the likelihood of users becoming and remaining employed. Firstly, most European countries have legislation that offers a measure of positive discrimination to people with a disability entering employment, either through a quota reserved for them in medium-sized and large workplaces and/or through a system of officers whose job it is to find suitable employment for disabled people.[39] However more often than not the state fails to ensure that the law is implemented in the spirit intended, as the lobbying power of people with disabilities is weaker than that of employers.

Secondly, in many cases users are likely to earn far less than the real wage within a work project, or are restricted to what have been termed 'therapeutic earnings', namely what one is allowed to earn without losing social security benefits. This level of payment is a disincentive to becoming a good worker, as it reminds user–workers of their dependency and powerlessness. Instead a more flexible system in which social security payments are suspended while people earn the usual wages for a job but are reinstated if the experiment fails, without a major reassessment and considerable delay, would be much more useful to both the individual and the state.

Employment projects

A range of employment initiatives have been created in Europe during the 1980s and the 1990s, not least because European Union antipoverty programmes and the Social Fund have enabled the channelling of resources into mental health services for this purpose only. The range includes sheltered workshops with traditional assembling jobs, employment training workshops where a variety of skills are taught (such as the use of computers, office skills, printing, picture framing, catering), supported work experiences, on-the-job training, social firms, work cooperatives, the use of high street employment placement agencies, and employment as a support worker.[40] The following stories highlight how work makes a difference to the lives of people who either continue to suffer from mental distress or have suffered from it in the past.

Katya is a pretty 20 year old living in Kiev. Her ability to paint and sculpt has been encouraged from early childhood by her parents. At the age of 15 she had her first schizophrenic breakdown, and was hospitalised for two years. Two more breakdowns followed, as well as hospitalisation periods. With her on the ward was Misha, whom she had known before. Katya and Misha have become close friends, as have their mothers. Both mothers were horrified by the physical conditions in the hospital, and by instances of the physical harming of patients. They started a relatives' group, the first in Ukraine, and were supported by a psychiatrist friend, who had contacts with American psychiatrists, based on his days in a Soviet labour camp. He introduced the two mothers to NAMI, the American relatives' organisation.

With a minimum amount of support from NAMI, and with growing support from the chief psychiatrist in Kiev, the relatives' group initiated a workshop outside the hospital that offers work making jewellery from porcelain, led by two artists. Both Katya and Misha work there quite happily. But Katya continues to destroy each beautifully finished product left with her. 'Rescued' products she is happy to leave untouched, and is pleased with being paid for her work. Financially the workshop is not viable.

Helen is 55 and is currently an instructor of office skills at a work project in central London. Not so long ago she was a patient, afraid to leave the house on her own and unable to make even the most banal decision. She was on medication for a long time, even though at one point there was no doubt as to the harm done by the medication, which was then changed. She initially went to another workshop as a means of leaving the house for a place that did not feel as degrading as a day centre. There she was introduced to more updated office skills than those she had possessed originally, and she began to feel more confident of her abilities as a worker. Helen moved to the current work project when she and the staff in the first workshop felt that she had learnt all she could there.

She appreciated the readiness of the staff of the new place to let her move at her own pace. Gradually, over eighteen months, she became sufficiently confident to be able to train other people who were newcomers to the project.

Elaine, the young manageress of the work project, insists on the necessity to separate 'patienthood' from 'being a worker', even for people on heavy medication who initially need ten minutes break for each five minutes of work.

In the following the focus is on work cooperatives as an example of an initiative that takes on board the new welfare climate, while continuing to provide opportunities for social role valorisation and self-management. Cooperatives now exist in a number of European countries, such as Britain, France,

Germany, Ireland, Italy and Switzerland. Productive activities include agriculture (Trieste, Pordenone, Turin), a variety of art forms (Trieste, Turin, Berlin), catering (Trieste), cleaning (Turin), electrical appliances (East Berlin), horse maintenance and riding lessons (Turin), printing (Dublin), furniture making (Trieste, Berlin), marketing (Parma), publishing (Trieste), toy making (Rome) and training in a variety of forms (Berlin, Manchester, Dublin).[41]

The cooperatives share the philosophy that:[42]

- work offers a positive strategy against marginalisation;
- people whose identities have been damaged and have been segregated do better in an environment that fosters solidarity;
- cooperatives encourage people to take responsibility not only for themselves, but also for others;
- cooperatives offer people an opportunity to move from dependency to interdependency;
- cooperatives engage in social production aimed at an improved redistribution of social justice;
- our most important resources are people and their creativity.

Cooperatives and all that they offer function within the world of production, where they have to compete with the not-so-free market. They are an example of quasi-markets *par excellence*, as they are created initially by welfare agencies for the benefit of service users.

The story told by one of the largest cooperatives in Europe, La Nuova Cooperativa (the New Cooperative) in Turin,[43] illustrates not only how a small cooperative can become a large enterprise, but also how market factors, politics, personalities, opportunities, successes and failures interact. The story is all the more remarkable because of the small number of non-users involved, namely ten out of two hundred members. Members do not earn the same, but there is a basic minimum hourly rate that everyone receives when they work. If absent, members do not lose their jobs; they are contacted, visited if necessary and persuaded to return. In principle members have an equal say in decision making, and most decisions are taken collectively.

The most important supportive components in terms of cooperative's everyday life include the work supervisors, the team with whom one works and decision-making meetings. Decision making is far from easy when a large number of people are involved, market conditions are unfavourable and the level of production is not very high. Some cooperatives have therefore opted to produce quality products rather than compete in mass production.

The financial cost of cooperatives is handled differently by different cooperatives. For example Trieste has opted not to focus on economic viability uses resources it managed to obtain when the hospitals closed. Pordenone – its geographical neighbour – is aiming to ensure that the cooperatives are financially viable, and has been reasonably successful in achieving this objective.[44] The financial contribution of the European Union (via its programmes against exclusion and marginalisation) has been crucial for all the European cooperatives.

The ultimate success of such schemes should be measured by the number of people who go on to work in ordinary organisations. However this indicator also depends on factors beyond the influence of the cooperatives or the individuals concerned (for example job availability), and therefore should not be used as the only criterion. Other positive outcomes include the number of people who successfully complete their training, people who remain to work within the programme, those who pursue further training, a reduction in the frequency of mental distress crise and mental distress symptomatology, an increase in well being and improved social functioning.

Angelo is 23 years old, a good looking young man with a hint of Down's Syndrome in his face. He lives with his mother in a small flat in an inner-city area in Trieste. I first met him in a restaurant, where he, his mother and an architect running a carpentry work cooperative were having supper and were engaged in what looked like an animated discussion. The restaurant was part of another work cooperative of the mental health services. I saw Angelo's work the following day when I visited the carpentry workshop. He specialised in painting the wooden surfaces of the post-modern furniture that others were making. His use of colour was stunning: vibrant, imaginative, adding a dimension to the futuristic furniture that made it warm, lively and fun to look at.

Angelo would be unlikely to succeed in an ordinary workplace, where often more than one ability is required and where speed would be asked for too. Angelo can be sulky, cheeky and explosive, but he can also be sweet and considerate, and he enjoys his work. The small cooperative, with seven workers only, seems ideal for him. It meets some of his needs for a supportive environment yet enables him to be productive and creative. In many other places Angelo would only be offered work in a sheltered workshop where packing or assembling jobs are the only options available.

Summary

The range of housing schemes mentioned above indicates that not only has it been accepted that people suffering from mental illness have the right to housing, but that their needs and wishes in this respect may differ. In Europe we have been successful in resettling people who have been in hospital for long periods of time, and less successful in resettling those who come through the acute admission route, especially those defined as homeless.

The range of initiatives concerning employment outlined above demonstrate that there are many ingenious ways of re-introducing the workplace to people who have suffered from mental distress, including severe distress, and of introducing others to employment for the first time. The need for ingenuity in this area is much greater than it is in relation to housing, and the initial financial investment can be quite limited. Investment in supporting and nurturing people so that they might know what they want and have a realistic appreciation of their abilities, which does not preclude having ambition and striving towards meeting their wishes, is necessary and often fruitful.

Are these projects viable? The answer depends in part on the definition of viability. New projects need to be nourished financially for a number of years and should not be expected to pay back the capital investment. After the first three years, given sound vocational advice, projects may begin to cover their expenditure. This has been the case in Germany, where a national organisation, the FAF (Forderung in Arbeitinitiativen und Firmenporjekten) provides advice on planning and funding.

Projects also need to be nourished in terms of public support and support to the managerial staff. Public support can take many forms, ranging from participating as a member of a project's management committee, to buying the product, to associating with the workers, to changing legislation on related social security issues.

Greater success in employment would ease the housing situation, as more service users, or ex-users, would be able to rent or buy their own housing, thus reducing public spending.

The recent creation of the umbrella organisation CEFEC (Confederation of European Firms, Employment Initiatives and Cooperatives for the Psychically Disabled) by the European Union, under the patronage of the commissioner for social affairs, promises better coordination and exchange of information among the different European schemes. This is a positive step in the right direction. However, without a fundamental change in the attitudes of professionals, sufferers, their relatives and the general public it will not be possible to put to good use what has been learned in Europe about employment opportunities over the last fifteen years. A readiness to think in terms of in and out of illness, and in, out and in again into employment, is a necessary condition for the success of the whole process of recovery from mental distress.

6
Changing Professional Roles and Identities

Louise's working day began at 9.00. She is stocky, her hair is cut short and she is dressed in jeans and a dowdy jacket. Only when she speaks do you identify her middle-class background. She walks slowly, looking at the entrances to the office buildings in the posh street in central London. Suddenly she spots Andy, a young man in his early 20s, sleeping in one of those entrances in a sleeping bag. Andy responds indifferently to her warm good morning greeting; he wants to continue to sleep. Both of them know that he has to move on soon, when the office workers start arriving. Louise offers to take Andy to a nearby cafe to have a cup of tea. Reluctantly he gets up and goes with her. While having tea they discuss what he is going to do today. Louise reminds him that they soon have to go to the hostel to see if his application has been successful, and then they will go to the Crypt, where he will see the GP, have lunch and participate in some of the group activities.

Described as 'a street worker' at a recent conference, Louise is a nurse specialising in young, homeless people who seem to be suffering from mental distress. She previously worked in a psychiatric ward in a general hospital. When asked about the links between her past and current posts she is more struck by the differences than the similarities, by her sense of liberation at not having to work routinely and on a ward, and the sense of well-earned satisfaction she feels when/if someone moves off the street into a more secure and stable way of living. She does not feel that everything in the hospital was bad; just that she can not see herself as being content with administering medication as a prime task.

Rocco dances enthusiastically with an older woman; then with a young one. After two hours of dancing (at a pre-Christmas party in the mental health centre) he is called hurriedly by the centre's receptionist to go out with a colleague on a home visit to someone who is reported to have been smashing everything within reach for the last half an hour. Rocco is a psychiatrist who directs a mental health centre in a deprived inner city area in southern Italy. He suggests that nothing in his studies at the medical school prepared him for his current post; that he had to work for a year in Trieste to rid himself of his training and past ways of working.

Richard is a lecturer in social work at a Dutch University. He is employing George, a well-known figure in the Dutch user movement, as a research officer in an action research project that is based in a psychiatric hospital and aimed at empowering the inpatients there. The hospital authorities are unhappy at present as a group of patients has become more rebellious than ever before, demanding more information and refusing to accept staff decisions at face value. For Richard and George this signifies the success of their project, but they are aware that their very presence in the hospital is at stake.

Despite the significant differences between the three examples outlined above, all three reflect how far-reaching the changes in professional roles, tasks and attitudes have become since 1980, at least for the professional workers described above.

The focus of the literature on professionalism ranges from issues of uniqueness in knowledge and skills as the base for claims for professional standing[1] to issues of power and gender.[2] When applied to mental health workers, the dominance of psychiatrists seems to combine successfully convincing all European societies that they have claims for unique knowledge with patriarchy, despite the fact that many women (and black men) work as psychiatrists, and despite the low status of psychiatry within medicine.

The emergence of community psychiatric nursing as a new subprofession in most European countries,[3] the new legal obligations of British social workers and the considerable increase in the number of unqualified workers within residential and daycare settings are some examples of the changes that have taken place in the traditional professional scene, of which the literature has hardly began to take account.

This chapter focuses on the implications of the developments in European mental health systems since 1980 to professional activities, knowledge, attitudes and self-image.

The considerable change in the structure of mental health services outlined in previous chapters implies a need for a parallel change in professional roles and identities, to enable professionals to work effectively within the new structures. However, as illustrated by descriptions of working with women and people from ethnic minorities as well as with continued care clients, the *content* of professional intervention within mainstream services has not changed that much. Therefore it is necessary to look at professional roles and identities from two parallel perspectives:

- the change aimed at, as reflected in the structural layer;
- the actual change in professional roles and identities.

Such an analysis should be followed by an understanding of *where* the gaps lie between intentions and realities, *what* has led to the creation and persistence of the gaps and *how* they can be bridged, if it is indeed desirable that these gaps should be bridged.

Professional roles consist of a series of tasks and responsibilities, usually mandated by the society in which the professionals are working on the basis of assumed professional expertise. In turn professional identity is based on professionals' claim to uniqueness in knowledge and skills.[4] Professional training and supervision, followed by an explicit set of ethical rules of conduct, are the main methods used to ensure that these claims have substance. The length of professional training in mental health varies from three years (after the completion of secondary education) to twelve, reflecting the agreed complexity of the roles and the wish to secure the internalisation of the training. Such an internalisation is crucial, as the decisions taken by mental health professionals concern a discretionary judgement of predictive risk, harm, strength and potential to recover and lead an ordinary life, taken against a background of uncertainty and insufficient knowledge.

The price of making the wrong decision can include murder, rape, arson, suicide, immense suffering, loss of opportunity to lead an ordinary life, and loss of freedom and dignity, affecting the identified sufferer, his/her relatives and society at large.

While professional identity is expected to be directly reflected in the role performed by the professional group and by individual professionals, a number of their tasks and responsibilities often evolve out of the organisational structure in which the professionals are functioning rather than out of their professional mandate as such. Therefore the possibility of conflicting demands arises, side by side with the likelihood of non-conflicting demands; professionals have to work their way around such eventualities. In sorting out conflicts and gaps in their practice, professional workers are expected to be guided by professional ethics first and foremost, yet the wish to protect one's job is understandably important to most people, as is loyalty to one's organisation. The delicate balancing act of loyalty to one's profession versus the organisation can become fragile at times, especially during periods of structural change and increasing organisational control.

In December 1985 Rocco, the Italian psychiatrist mentioned above, showed me round the psychiatric facilities of the general hospital in B, a southern Italian city. After visiting the family therapy unit, with its one-way screen and plush furniture, he took me to the admission ward. A good few minutes were needed to open the iron door to the ward, an extremely bare environment in comparison with the family therapy unit. He went ahead of me to have a chat with a client from his area who had been admitted the day before. Suddenly Rocco shouted at the top of his voice: 'remove it, or I'll do it myself, you bastards'. I rushed in to the small room to find that the client was chained to the bed. Rocco was much more shocked than the client, and angrier too. The nursing officer came hurriedly, explaining to Rocco that the patient had been agitated the previous night. Rocco remained unconvinced, and simply said to the nursing officer that they had five minutes in which to remove the chain themselves or he would do it – or they could face the alternative, which would be a formal complaint to the police and health authorities of the illegal arrest of a citizen. The nursing officer complied without uttering a further word.

Rocco continued to fume as we left the ward, telling me that this was but one example of what he had to guard against and expect from those opposing the change in the Italian psychiatric system.

Freedom to care[5] is a new British organisation aimed at supporting professional 'whistle-blowers', namely professionals who publicly speak out against the practices of their organisation. They are often disciplined and/or dismissed by their employers on the ground of disloyalty to the organisation, rather than on the ground of not speaking the truth. The organisation claims that the number of such cases has recently increased, as the government – still the biggest employer of mental health professionals – and the newly established health trusts (looked at in Chapter 1) formally prevent professionals from voicing their criticisms in public. In turn the employers claim that there are satisfactory internal channels for criticisms to be taken up. The rule of thumb is that the less stable the contractual basis of employment becomes, the less likely it is that insiders will speak up for fear of being blocked for promotion or dismissed, as well as being fearful of rocking the boat of which they are a part.

Few examples of successful whistle blowing, exist in the context of mental health services where success is measured by improved standards of care on the one hand and by the whistle blower retaining his/her post on the other. Mrs Sue Machin recently lost her appeal against dismissal from her post as social worker at Ashworth special hospital after making allegations of maltreatment by workers–prison officers in that institution. Despite the fact that the inquiry committee set up to investigate these allegations found them to be true and recommended changes in the everyday practices there, the industrial tribunal found her guilty of passing internal information to an outside body. Her case demonstrates that the legal power of employers is stronger than the moral power of exposing wrongdoing to stop unacceptable professional conduct.

At the other end of the spectrum are professionals against whom unjustified allegations have been made in an attempt to get rid of them because they were perceived as 'trouble makers', or simply did not toe the line required by the bosses. This process can take years, with a considerable financial, social and psychological price to pay.

Dr R., whose paper I heard at a conference in Lisbon in June 1993, has been reinstated after a five-year suspension without pay from his post of director of a psychiatric hospital in northern Portugal after being accused of malpractice by some of the nurses working in the hospital. He had to bring the Ministry of Health to court to prove his innocence, and then had to wait for two years to be reinstated and financially compensated for the lost years. During these five years his wife, a doctor herself, was the only breadwinner. One can only imagine the difficulties that she too had to live with. Not surprisingly, Dr R. has chosen not to return to the same hospital. It is not known what has happened to those who made the allegations.

An important issue about which we lack information is what happens to professionals who have not followed ethical rules of behaviour and have been found out, dismissed or demoted. The paucity of research into the ethical dilemmas faced by mental health professionals reflects the complexity of the professional role and identity, as well as social apprehension about looking too closely at this uncomfortable issue.

The major structural changes in the 1980s and 1990s have consisted of:

- The transfer of services from hospital to community bases, together with a greater emphasis on reducing the duration of admissions and attempting to prevent as many of them as possible.
- Closer multidisciplinary work than in the past, and on a more equal footing.
- The introduction of a multisectored service system, in which the monopoly of the public sector has been broken and private not-for-profit and for-profit organisations now dominate areas such as sheltered housing, nursing homes, employment projects and psychotherapy.
- A more dominant management component and a more managerial ethos – as distinct from professional ethos – has come to the fore.[6]
- The more vocal presence of user and carer groups in at least four European countries (Britain, Germany, Italy, the Netherlands), as discussed in Chapter 4. This is reflected in considerable criticisms being voiced on the subject of professional intervention.
- All of this has taken place against a background of reduced public expenditure and constraints on financial and human resources.

Applied to professional roles, this has meant the following. First, to an extent the changes were/are a reflection of self-critique or critiques expressed by others of professional activities prior to the policy change.

Second, the range of assessments to be made, interventions to be offered and discretionary decisions to be made has shifted to reflect the attempt to keep people in the community and away from hospitals, and/or to ensure the reduction of admission periods. Knowledge of formal and informal resources in the community has become more important than ever before.[7] Assessing the abilities and strengths of clients, their informal carers and their environment has become more central than before, and in a number of professional practices it has been discovered for the first time that this constitutes useful knowledge.[8]

Third, more professionals are working in community-based facilities than ever before, and fewer are working in psychiatric hospitals, psychiatric wards in general hospitals and secure units.

Fourth, working in the community implies working in a smaller unit than before, with fewer colleagues and at times with no other colleague of the same discipline. Both the controlling and the comforting aspects of the large institution have therefore disappeared. Hence professionals have to get used to different controlling and comforting mechanisms, or invent them (for example no canteen, no patients to do cleaning jobs, no big Christmas party, no allocation of uniform clothing, no set times to have lunch/tea/coffee breaks).

Fifth, workers now interact daily with members of other disciplines, who may also be their line managers. Major decisions are taken in the multidisciplinary team. This may entail talking more regularly to members of other disciplines, obtaining more knowledge of the other discipline and its ways of working, reconsidering one's beliefs and myths about them, creating new alliances and at times personal friendships. Alternatively it may mean working with incompatible perspectives and the tension that such a coexistence generates, without the physical buffers available in a large institution.

The level of competition for power increases as the representatives of the different disciplines have a more equal say, but they may also wish to secure/increase the power of their own discipline. Alternatively disciplinary boundaries may become less important than they were before, and the internal team becomes the core of cohesion and identity for its members. This usually takes place where traditional forms of professional practice are open to critical discussion.

Sixth, there are now more clearly defined managerial rules and professional targets (task centred, behavioural, care management) following the adoption of conceptual and practice models that facilitate clarity of targets and the discarding of models that fail to facilitate such clarity. However this change is often accompanied by a huge increase in paperwork and a reduction in both professional autonomy and the time spent with clients.

This outcome is more typical of countries in which the government was driving force behind structural change, and does not seem to apply to those countries in which structural change came out of professional demands.

Seventh, the politicisation of the professional workforce is another outcome accompanying structural change, either at the motivational base for the change (Italy) or as a reaction to imposed change (Britain, France, Germany).[9]

Eighth, more managers have been introduced to key positions in health and social services than before in Britain, symbolising a belief in the managerial ethos that closely follows American beliefs in the usefulness of applying a business ethos to public sector services. Many of them came with no knowledge of mental health and distress, but were keen to implement the structural changes and to demonstrate their own usefulness and that of the managerial ethos. From the early 1980s professionals began to join the managerial class.

The assumption of the universality of knowledge of organisations is widespread in the First World, as is belief in the applicability of knowledge culled from business-oriented structures to non-profit public sector services. At a certain level of abstraction such applicability exists, as we are dealing with human resources. Yet at another level the similarity is only skin-deep, and the application becomes an attempt to distort the character of one organisational structure to fit the ideological convictions of another such structure.

Ninth, a small number of key professionals have been empowered at the expense of others and – so far – at the expense of service users in controlling vital resources, for example the control over budgets now available to British GPs, who can buy specialist services and a variety of social services if they so choose. A somewhat more modest control is available to care management budget holders, who can decide on packages of services to people with severe disabilities, including mental illness. The legislation on care management stipulates consultation with clients and relatives, but does not specify what is meant by such consultation.

So far the findings are that GPs who have opted to be budget holders are thrilled by the opportunities opened to them in accessing and controlling specialist care.[10] Those who have opted not to do so argue that their patients are discriminated against by being put at the end of the queue because the GP is not a budget holder. It is relevant to note that the research did not include the views of patients and their relatives on whether they are consulted more now than in the past, whether the GPs' decisions reflected their choices or ignored them, and whether services are provided more quickly and effectively than in the past.

Tenth, many more unqualified care workers are now employed in Those mental health services where it is deemed that there is less urgent need for discretionary decisions, such as in residential and day care.[11] This relates in part to the growing presence of private sector operators in this field, where for cost reduction purposes fewer professionals are employed and when employed are used sparingly, for sessional contributions rather than as full-time employees. This preference also relates to the view that support for ordinary living is best provided by non-professional, more 'ordinary' people.[12]

Some of the implications of this policy have been outlined in Christine McCourt Perring's study of three newly established group homes for resettled long-stay patients from hospitals due for closure.[13] Negative aspects include care staff being overdependent on the medical model, partly for purposes of playing it safe and partly because they have insufficient knowledge about alternative approaches, as well as an overriding sense that their lack of knowledge prevents them from carrying out the job properly.

Eleventh, users and relatives' views are being heard more than they were before, and some user-led or relative-led initiatives are to be found.[14] However on the whole these views are not followed up if they imply a departure from the accepted political or professional wisdom. For example British service users have expressed in no uncertain terms their wish and need for counselling. But counselling is presently perceived as 'politically incorrect' because it is more expensive than medication, it often requires an unspecified duration, and the targets to be achieved are not easy to define and measure.

Those professionals who are ready to listen to users are likely to find themselves in a difficult position if they follow users' views and discard traditional professionally accepted approaches.

V. is a psychiatrist involved in setting up the first care management and employment project for young people suffering from mental illness in Slovenia. The project is funded by the Ministry of Welfare, and has not been supported by the Ministry of Health, her formal employer. She is currently on maternity leave, and is thus working in a voluntary, unpaid capacity. V. is worried that when her leave ends she will have to choose between her secure post in a psychiatric hospital and the less secure work at the new not-for-profit organisation, provided the latter manages to find the additional funding for her post. At the same time, she is the *only* psychiatrist in Slovenia to be involved in this type of innovative work. At a recent meeting with the director of the Slovenian psychiatric services her work was presented as a positive example of new developments in Slovenian psychiatry; yet any attempt to carry out this work *within* the structure of the formal system has been rejected to date. What would you have done in her place?

Working with users and carers in an empowering way often requires a shift in attitudes, knowledge and skills, especially in those instances where the users and carers are encouraged to work in their own groups. Workers have to let group members make the main decisions and implement them, while providing advice and some of the tools and means required. Providing *background* support rather than *foreground* help is a new experience to many mental health professionals, as is letting service users get on with the task. Milroy and Hennelly[15] have proposed that full empowerment will be achieved when professionals become redundant not due to cuts in public expenditure but because their expertise is no longer needed. Working towards becoming redundant has an ironical twist to it, highlighting the centrality of the process of power being *given away* by professionals and taken by users and carers in the implementation of empowerment.

Few of us are unreservedly pleased about giving away power. This assertion may seem strange, as professionals have always had to rely on the client – and his/her relatives – to both opt for changes and implement them, given that the changes expected in relation to mental distress are often at the psychological, social and behavioural levels. Yet in the one-to-one worker and client encounter the power of the professional worker to tilt the client's perceptions in the direction of the worker's views is considerable, even – or especially – at the preconscious, emotional level, where rational argument alone is often insufficiently persuasive. The attitudes, knowledge and skills that need to be fostered as preconditions for empowerment happening are encapsulated by the social role valorisation approach[16], briefly outlined in Chapter 2.

Nearly all of the writings and work carried out under this umbrella framework provide ample examples of responses to the basic question that has to be remembered at all time as the yardstick by which to measure whether what I, as a professional, am doing is good enough: would I like to use this service for myself or a friend? Brandon[17] and Segal,[18] who come from two different professional traditions (social role valorisation and psychoanalysis) yet share a similar value base, have highlighted that the core of the enabling professional relationships lies in a humanistic response to the pain the client is suffering from, where the professional remembers intuitively that she/he too is not immune to such suffering, as well as remembering that the service user has abilities that should be encouraged to be fully made use of, and rights not only to the best service she/he may need, but also to *make their own informed decisions*.

Given these dimensions, the role of the professional is being redefined from one who knows best to one who:

- listens to the client;
- shares the pain;
- learns from the client;
- shares knowledge and information with the client in a way that the client can understand;
- intermediates at times with other agencies and people on behalf of the client;
- helps to create new, informal and flexible services if these are needed;
- indicates the advantages and disadvantages of proposed solutions, but leaves it to the client to make the final decision;
- supports the client in identifying her/his strengths and weaknesses and developing her/his abilities, including the skills

required for decision making, thus enlarging the range of coping and reflective strategies open to the person.

Twelfth, quality assurance measures have been introduced in a few European countries, such as instituting complaints and appeal procedures, allowing clients access to their own files, inspecting standards, providing written and monitored contracts, introducing periodical consultation and encouraging regular feedback by users (Britain, the Netherlands, the Scandinavian countries).[19] However relatively few clients and carers exploit these possibilities, mainly because of instilled fear of the repercussions of expressing criticism, and doubts that complaining will lead to constructive measures being taken to change the situation.

A recent but small example of introducing quality assurance to a residential setting[20] highlights the importance of the process of involving users in such an introduction. It demonstrates that for the residents to *own* the quality assurance procedure it is vital that they be given the opportunity to voice their doubts about the staff's sincerity in introducing it, as well as for the staff to leave it in the hands of the residents.

Finally, an increasing number of professionals have transferred to private not-for-profit or for-profit agencies. This relates in part to a wish to retain autonomy and a good income, and in part because that is where the new job opportunities lie. Thus a larger number of newcomers are to be found in the non-public sector because of a lack of jobs within the public sector.

Where health services are mediated by insurance companies (as is the case in Germany and the Netherlands) more *office psychiatrists* are to be found, almost taking us back to pre-national health service times. To a certain extent this is a paradoxical move, as office psychiatrists are unlikely to be interested in or knowledgeable about community facilities and networks, and thus provide a narrower range of intervention than the structural changes are aimed at. Yet this narrow range fulfills another requirement of the change, namely targeted, time-limited, cheap intervention.

How did mental health professionals respond to these wide-ranging changes, which represent a watering down of the more fundamental changes hoped for? Before attempting to provide some answers to this question, it is important to remember the specific challenges that face mental health workers. Elsewhere[21] I have outlined the fragility, the fascination and the vulnerability entailed in mental health work. These characteristics are accompanied by workers employing coping strategies that enable them to live with the suffering of others, the duality of providing both care and control, and the need to make crucial decisions within a wide margin of uncertainty. Julia Segal,[22] a psychologist working in a not-for-profit organisation in West London that focuses on people suffering from multiple sclerosis, has gone further in indicating the pain experienced by the professional, the wish to be omnipotent but the inability to be so, and envy of clients over qualities and experiences that the worker feels she/he has missed so far in her/his private life.

Working with survivors of sexual abuse perhaps magnifies the impact of work experiences on professionals. The urgent wish to be rescuer, redeemer and restorer becomes clearer than in other instances of mental health work.[23] Empathy with the survivors as against loathing the perpetrators or the larger category of those perceived as being 'silent' partners to the abuse (notably mothers wives) is also more upfront in this instance than in other types of mental distress work. So must be the level of disappointment when the work does not proceed as positively as wished by the worker, which is more often the case than not. All of this is magnified when issues of ethnicity and racism come into it, as they do in cases of sexual abuse within ethnic minority families.[24] Support for professionals working in the areas of mental health and sexual abuse is therefore a crucial issue.

Responses to the structural changes are constantly mediated against the background of these considerations and coping strategies. At this specific juncture they are also influenced by the sense of failure and frustration experienced by many professionals as a generalised reaction to the radical changes, and the sense of excitement and positive challenge felt by a minority across the mental health professions.[25]

The latter applied on a grand scale in Italy during the 1970s and the early 1980s, when a vocal minority group of professionals mobilised a radical restructuring of the mental health system, bolstered by strong public support yet without the active support of the government. The value base and the political message and analysis of that far-reaching reform were relatively clear. The very existence of an upfront, explicit message has been referred to as 'ideological' by those professionals who continue to believe that professional activity (and scientific inquiry) exist without a *biased* value base, and without political connotations.[26] This very British position is not shared anywhere else in Europe, even though European professionals can be heard muttering that they wish they could be left to their own devices, free from interference by their country's appointed politicians.

The value base of the Italian reformers included treating people with mental illness as citizens, focusing on the damage done to them and *to the rest of us* by segregation, and on the need to undo that damage. This was believed in at a time when evidence for the success of resettlement in the community, dismantling psychiatric hospitals and establishing a community-based service system was largely non-existent. Therefore leaping in this direction was a bold act of faith and experimentation, with considerable risk attached. Instead of proven experiments, the knowledge base was constructed eclectically from personal experiences of solidarity and social action from British social psychiatry and British anti-psychiatry, from French existentialism, from the Italian socialist tradition, and from the pragmatic lessons of actually working with the long-term residents and staff of psychiatric hospitals.[27]

The overall success of the Italian reform in closing hospitals and establishing community mental health services attests to the usefulness of the approach of its initiators. At the same time it depended heavily on continuous good will and a readiness to invest personally and communally without the back-up support of either proven knowledge or existing structures. This has meant a very uneven national development, with no means of quality assurance. It was/is a matter of luck whether you – or your relative – live in an area with good or bad services. Of necessity, it has also implied a measure of trial and error, which perhaps could not have been avoided.

That the reformers have used so little of their own knowledge of psychiatry within the reform process reflects the poverty of psychiatry in enabling and generating reform. The conceptual changes introduced as part of the reform included:[28]

- The value of people working for an organisation, rather than of the organisation first.
- The importance of organisational structures above professional intervention methods.
- The importance of collective action as a motivator of users, professionals, the community.
- Rediscovering continued care clients as people worthy of professional and human attention.
- Bringing to the fore the abilities for positive change that were suppressed within continuing care clients during their many years of hospitalisation.
- Exposing in a forceful way the harm done by long-term hospitalisation.
- Beginning the search for a new professional identity.

Despite all these innovations, when looked at from the perspective of the 1990s the Italian reformers have been unsuccessful in changing the basic principles of psychiatry and its knowledge base. It is as if the considerable success of the reform has left the knowledge base of Italian – and European – psychiatry untouched.

While continuing to practice in an innovative way in some areas, the achievements of the reform are now grouped under the heading 'psychiatric rehabilitation' as a sub-branch of general psychiatry, focusing on individual users and not on the context in which they live, work or are being treated.[29] With few exceptions, the focus on reforming society and reforming professional work and thinking has been largely forgotten. The research methods used are no better than anywhere else in mainstream European psychiatry, and in many cases methods used elsewhere are copied without sufficient thought being given to their usefulness.

In attempting to understand why this has happened, it seems to me that:

- The Italian reforming psychiatrists have continued to see themselves as psychiatrists and to view the contribution of medicine as largely beneficial and therefore not in need of fundamental change. Furthermore they wished to be part of mainstream psychiatry, rather than continuing to be splendidly isolated but without giving up their value commitments.

Changing Professional Roles and Identities 175

- The pragmatic focus prevented an equal investment in a conceptual reshaping process.
- The other professional groups, weaker in social status and cultural standing, accepted the leadership of the psychiatrists until fairly late in the day, when the psychologists within the reform movement began to develop their more distinct contribution. Nurses in Italy have not yet developed a distinct professional identity, which perhaps has prevented them from adding their contribution.[30]
- The preference for a unified professional mental health worker, which made sense in view of the considerable overlap of roles and tasks in the earlier period of the Italian reform, seems to have evaporated since the late 1980s. A return to disciplinary divisions has been evident in some of the regions (for example, Tuscany). Even where this has not taken place, too much power continues to be concentrated in the hands of psychiatrists.
- The majority of Italian mental health professionals who initially opposed the reform have not changed their conceptual background, even when they have changed their methods of work and some components of their value base. Organic psychiatry, psychoanalysis and family therapy have as strong a fellowship as before.
- The message of collectively empowering users and relatives has barely been taken up across Italy, despite the initial focus on collective action and empowering individual service users, and despite the more recent stimulating initiatives around user participation and mutual support in places such as Imola, Prato and Trieste.[31]

Reformers in France have focused instead on exploring:[32]

- The intricate relationship between being entitled to benefits by registering as disabled and thus being committed to adopting the identity of a disabled person, rather than the identity of an able person who has a disability.
- The interaction between social control of our private lives (for example sexuality, the family) and approaches to madness and to working with people exhibiting madness.
- Psychoanalytical approaches combined with structuralist and discourse analysis influences.

British reformers do not speak in one voice, but are split into three camps:

- Those who believe in the centrality of organisational and administrative change and have wholeheartedly adopted US approaches to public administration, which are based on profit- making organisational logic.[33] Professional interventions within such a framework are perceived as just one of a number of possible operational methods, and a rather costly one at that.
- Those who have adopted the normalisation and social role valorisation approach, often adding to it the focus on user involvement, and a critique of Wolfensberger's Christian, male, white, middle-class orientation.[34]
- Those who continue to believe that the best approach to restructuring mental health services is through a rehabilitative model, best achieved by behavioural methods at the individual client and relative level.[35]

There does not seem to be a conflict between the first and the third approach, but for some there is a degree of incompatibility between the first and the second approach, as well as between the second and third frameworks. The debate is dominated by disagreements on the value of the government-led reorganisation of the welfare system.

Some of those who have adopted the social role valorisation approach have argued that the new managerial approach and the privatisation of welfare services offer a valuable new opportunity for the implementation of principles such as choice, and need-led and wishes-led services, including the client having control over who is hired – and fired – to work for him/her.[36] Others have been more sceptical about the ability of a privatised service, ruled by market forces, to offer good quality.

Within the brokerage approach in particular the place of professional intervention is seen as limited to specified services, and the less it is required the better.[37] This preference has developed out of the critique of professional input and the assumption that its paternalism is inherent and cannot be avoided.

The *resettlers* consist of two major groups: those who work within the hospital on the planned process of preparing for resettlement, and those who take over the work with the resettled people once they are outside.[38] Unlike the Italian process,

Changing Professional Roles and Identities 177

little continuity from the first group to the second seems to have been planned for or happened by chance. The inside resettlers focus on assessment and planning services, purchasing and contracting, and at times will be part of the management committee of a new service in the community. Once the assessment has been carried out and the plans drawn, they call in the implementers, often unqualified paid care staff from not-for profit or for-profit organisations, to prepare the long-stay residents for the move to the outside.

This type of work illustrates that the split between purchasers and providers was not created by the NHS and Community Care Act of 1990 (described in Chapter 1), but is rooted further back. It also highlights the fact that the psychological, relational and networking tasks have been relegated into less desirable elements by the new managerial class and the ruling political group. With this relegation, most non-medical professional input has been relegated too.

> J. is one of the few who have followed the process through. A trained occupational therapist who worked in a day centre, she became a member of one of the first wave of resettlement teams. Initially working in a hospital, and later partly in the hospital and partly in the community, she is now the manager of a community-based care management programme for a subgroup of people now defined as 'difficult to place'. Her team consists of professionals from a variety of disciplines, united by their wish to escape their previous place of work – perceived by them as stifling initiative and failing both clients and workers – into a more creative and flexible setting. Not surprisingly the specific care management approach adopted by them is based on the strength model described in Chapter 4.

Slovenia offers us an interesting example of the mixed impact of its Alp-Adria neighbours (Italy and Austria), the European Union (which supported a major training initiative in mental health there between 1990 and 1994) and Britain (a partner in the EU programme). Slovenian reformers have come mainly from the fields of social work and psychology, and are as yet to engage sufficient psychiatrists and nurses for the reform process to gather momentum. Influenced by British, French and Italian reformers, they selected those aspects that appealed to them within their understanding of the post-communist Slovenian context.

T. is a lecturer in psychology at the university, and at times a patient of the local psychiatric clinic. Since completing her Tempus-funded post-qualifying community mental health training, doing her fieldwork in Italy, she has coordinated an advocacy project that provides users with legal representation and advocacy in their dealings with professionals, usually psychiatrists. Most of those requesting advocacy come from the well-educated, young user group. The legal and medical establishment are astounded at what they perceive to be an affront.

N. is a social worker who used to work in a general social work centre. Together with V., a psychiatrist who used to work in the major psychiatric hospital of the country, N. has established a new day centre. The first of its kind in Slovenia, it offers a rehabilitation programme to people hospitalised for a mental illness crisis, with a work-orientated programme for some of them. N. and V. learned about such possibilities in London.

G. is a social worker who volunteered to work with the Croatian refugees who swamped Slovenia in 1991, only to be replaced after a few months by refugees from Bosnia. She has become director of the refugees service in Ljublijana. This is a rather unenviable job as the refugees live an ex-army barracks, are not allowed to work or study with the Slovenians, are anxious and depressed, and are not particularly liked by the ordinary Slovenian on the street.

G. spent most of 1993–4 in search of money, and seems to have been too exhausted to lead a normal life for the last two years. She has built up a service where both volunteers and professionals are dedicated to improving the living standard and quality of life of the refugees. It is difficult to estimate how many mental illness crisis have been prevented by this work, as against how many refugees have been scarred for life by their experiences.

M. is working for the Ministry of Welfare, quietly spearheading the new understanding and investment in mental health services within the ministry.

T., N., G. and M. are representatives of some of the services on offer, and many more innovative services have been developed as recently as this year by a small number of equally dedicated psychologists and social workers.

The Slovenian reformers have also had a go at developing their own critical understanding of approaches to mental health and rehabilitation. They are sceptical of British superpragmatism and of the too congratulatory normalisation approach, adopting elements from Foucault in criticising it.

Despite all these achievements, impressive in part because they have been established in such a short time by a relatively small group of people with few resources, the mental health system in Slovenia is yet to change at its core. Its psychiatrists – leaders are holding out against any move to the community. Most Slovenian politicians are largely as uninterested in mental health issues as they were before. However a minority within the Ministry of Welfare, influenced by the reformer group, are now ready to sponsor the new not-for-profit mental health services mentioned above.

Thus the Slovenian example highlights the wide-ranging potential for innovation in mental health services that even a small group of dedicated people can achieve. It also illustrates well the limitations imposed by the combined effect of the power differential within mental health systems and vested interests in preventing such innovations from taking place.

Changes in professional power, roles and identities

J. and her team have utilised the structural changes in the mental health system to create an island of innovative practice. The island has benefited them as individuals too, as it has enabled them to modify considerably their previous way of working to methods they prefer, *and* it has added to their power as professionals. Their power is enhanced in part because as care managers they have become the gatekeepers and purchasers of services, and in part because of the special status of the project as a new innovation. This project provides an interesting example of how empowering users and divesting oneself of professional power in the process of doing so may also entail the acquisition of new professional power.

Another example, referred to in Chapter 1, is the considerable increase in the legal power of British mental health social workers since 1983 in their role as approved social workers (ASWs). As ASWs they have a major say in whether or not a person should be compulsorily admitted to hospital, in looking for the least restrictive alternative environment, in acting as the person's guardian, and in coordinating the process of discharge from hospital to the community of people who had been compulsorily admitted.[39]

A considerable amount of time and resources are given to training ASWs and updating their initial training. However most of training is focused on risk assessment and sensitivity to cultural differences,[40] and only a fraction is given to promoting mental health, social role valorisation of service users, mental health policies and innovation in mental health. There is evidence to suggest that while traditionally unhappy with the controlling function that the role of the ASW entails, at present mental health social workers are more pleased than displeased with this role because of the power it gives them. This represents a major shift from the past, and from the stated preference of mental health social workers to offer on-going counselling rather than focusing on assessment.[41] It may well be that the sense of power inferiority in relation to other professions, notably psychiatrists, and the poor media image that mental health social workers have in Britain makes social workers feel better about this relatively new source of power, regardless of what it in fact implies.

Jones and Poletti[42] have suggested that Italian professionals have been through a process of deprofessionalisation by undertaking the task of supporting people in ordinary living, which does not require professional training (for example shopping with them, going for outings). The Italians' response is that they have been through a process of *reprofessionalisation*[43] in which they have moved away from rigid to flexible ways of working, including more participatory methods of response that equalise power differences.

The much larger number of unqualified staff working now in mental health services brings to a head the issue of the current and future role of professionals. The interpretation of the role of the care manager as an assessor and purchaser in some British social services departments versus the interpretation of this role as assessor and continuing service provider in some other such departments highlights further the centrality of this issue.

The changing roles and identities of professionals are yet to attract the in-depth research and understanding they deserve. One of the very few studies to look at the interface between structural changes and professional roles and identifies has focused on the reactions of three teams of social workers to the closure of the psychiatric hospital in which they worked during the middle and final phases of the closure.[44] It highlights a process in which workers who believed in such a closure and in the value of community living for most people suffering from mental illness have been alienated from the restructuring process and from actively contributing to it. Instead they have become cynical about the likelihood of the success of closure and resettlement, as well as about the potential for good multidisciplinary collaboration. Furthermore the process has not led them to reexamine constructively their professional role and identity, but has made them more defensive about these aspects and has imposed further bureaucratic constraints on their professional autonomy. While putting clients' well-being and respect at the top of their professional agenda, they have demonstrated little interest in – and knowledge about – the participation of users and carers.

The process of alienation is rooted in the way their own organisation (social services) and the umbrella organisation (the hospital, run by the health service) have gone about involving professional frontline workers in the change process. This process is characterised by a lack of real, non-lip-service consultation and participation by a highly skilled group of workers in a *value-shared* restructuring. Thus in the name of managerial efficiency, focused as it is on the usefulness of hierarchical management, a major source of agents for active change has been squandered.

Pertaining to imposing change on professionals, Britain is not exceptional. Apart from Italy in the 1970s and early 1980s, for most of the time in most European countries such attempts to involve workers have been replaced by prescriptions from above as to what workers should be doing from now on.

Elsewhere[43] I have described how the Italian reformers went about involving the people working in the hospitals, turning most of them into active partners in the process of both hospital closure and developing mental health services in the community. The same time-honoured principles of involving people as worthwhile contributors known to us from community development, action research, political activities and profitable but intelligent private enterprise operate in relation to professionals as they do in relation to users and carers.[46] The majority of European mental health workers remain oblivious to the need for solidarity, beyond its value as a self-help tool. In turn self-help is not something they would themselves recommend or participate in, but one that – at most – they would allow social workers and nurses to engage in.

With a few notable exceptions (such as the Dutch community social work centres), psychiatrists, psychologists, nurses, occupational therapists and social workers know little about the neighbourhoods in which they work beyond the level of formal organisations and are not trained to get to know them, and consequently are handicapped when they look for an alternative to formal services. Likewise they do not know how to approach users as a collective, how to tap into their knowledge of the neighbourhood or the value of professional intervention.

Most of them cannot see the point of finding out what their clients want beyond the individual level, and are sure that the spokespersons of the user movement are not 'true' representatives as they have not been 'properly elected', as if the representatives of any professional association have been elected and are truly representative of their constituency. They are then shocked and dismayed when the negative views of users and carers are made public, and attempt to dismiss such messages as unreliable and invalid. Even knowledge of policies and new legislation is perceived as knowledge of technicalities and tasks, with no place given to the need to understand and know the context in which specific policies are rooted, or even the inherent contradictions between and within specific policies.

The lack of fundamental change in the professional practice of many workers, the dismissal of the positive significance of the structural changes and the tendency to view all changes as negative almost *a priori*, also reflect a training deficiency. In turn the lack of preparation to be an active change agent reflects on professional values. The latter continue to be firmly rooted in the value of a clinical model, methodologically based on medicine and the natural sciences, in which the professional contribution is assumed to be based on discretionary decision making that is not context-bound but 'objective' and 'universal'. Knowledge of the context does not qualify as either objective or universal. Consequently even new professionals such as community psychiatric nurses want to become proficient in counselling methods, but not in social intervention. Members of older professions such as psychiatry treat the demand for new knowledge as essentially out of place.

The focus on pragmatic knowledge, shared by many European professionals and the managers of business organisations, is often useful. However it is also a further hindrance to contextual knowledge or to dwelling on ethical questions. The latter become seen as luxuries that cannot be afforded. While these trends may be stronger in some countries than others, they threaten to turn the achievements of the structural change into a mere relocation exercise, lacking in substance (as has happened in the United States).[47]

Handling potential and actual violence

A further, newly emerging threat to the structural changes lies in the reemphasis on the risk of violence by users. So far this has emerged as a central theme only in Britain, as already mentioned in Chapters 1 and 4. Fostered by a general panic over law and order issues, and especially by the media's inflammatory treatment of the violent acts of a tiny minority of psychiatric patients (looked at in Chapter 7), the sense of panic has reached training organisations and workers alike.

While attacks on workers should be prevented, it is doubtful whether the focus on assumed risk from clients and on restraining techniques offer the best means of achieving such aims. It is likely that such an approach will only heighten the sense of alienation and lead to an escalation of violent reactions. This may be the case due to several omissions: looking at the contribution the specific setting makes to the level of frustration exhibited by the client, including frustration of workers, and working on the reasons behind the violence are omitted from consideration by the narrow focus on restraint techniques. This particular response reminds us of the violence-tainted atmosphere that prevailed in the old psychiatric hospitals, which women patients tell us is still prevailing today in psychiatric wards in general hospitals and in special hospitals.[48]

Further professional responses

The division between the reformers and the majority of the professionals who are treating the reforms as a fashion that will go away like any other fashion, seems to exist in most Northern and Southern European countries. The majority have opted for further specialisation as a response to the changes, often along the divide of either clinical – somatic psychiatry, or clinical – psychological psychiatry. Within these divisions there are further qualitative differences, such as between those who have developed cognitive behavioural methods and those who have explored psychoanalytical psychotherapy. These two psychological schools of thought have expanded their expertise at more than one level and with more than one client group. Thus cognitive behaviourists have begun to pay much more attention to concepts and not only to habit formation, to continued care clients and people whose behaviour is defined as 'challenging', to a reevaluation of traditional diagnosis (as described in Chapter 2), and to cross the boundaries between mental illness and learning difficulties.[49]

Some psychoanalysts have developed their ways of working by reforming psychotherapy with women and members of ethnic minorities, as described in Chapter 3. Others have turned to working with sexual abuse survivors, despite Freud's assertion that such abuse is all in the mind. Still others have begun to offer non-classical psychoanalytic psychotherapy to people defined as having learning difficulties, who seem to respond positively to being treated as a human being with a respected depth of feelings. More refined ways of working with whole families have been developed, paying attention to gender issues within the context of family therapy.[50]

CAT (cognitive analytic therapy) is another new direction in psychotherapy that aims to combine elements of cognitive and behavioural therapy with psychoanalytic dimensions.[51] This is a form of short-term psychotherapy for individuals experiencing a range of difficulties, including some that most of the more traditional psychotherapists tend either not to engage in or are unsuccessful with. In a recent publication Ryle and Beard[52] describe working with a woman diagnosed as having a borderline personality disorder, who moved from rage to depression and self-harm. After 26 sessions (much longer than the usually time limit of 12 sessions) she was able to face her painful memories without this leading to a bout of anger or depression, to confront important people in her life in a way that was productive for both sides, and to find the strength to see the positive within herself without wallowing in self-pity or making unrealistic demands on others, while making realistic demands and expecting these to be met.

This high level of innovation reflects the creativity existing within current professional groups. That it is divorced from the structural changes is regrettable, but it is intriguing and requires an explanation. It seems to me that the explanation lies in the earlier divorce between politicians and planners on the one side, and the professionals on the other, as well as in the internal schism within the professions, where because truth is impossible to establish with sufficient certainty, faith in a total system replaces certainty.

Unless we find a way of putting together the different elements highlighted above, of reducing the level of inflexibility that the changed organisational systems seem to have brought with them, and of turning most professionals into active participants in the change process, we run a serious risk of retaining the structural changes as empty shells.

7
A Scandalous Category: Media Representations of People Suffering from Mental Illness

The importance of the media in shaping public opinion is taken for granted these days. However understanding its impact on the public, and on politicians, professionals, users and their relatives, is facilitated little by merely repeating this belief. Furthermore, what is usually taken for granted is the assumed unidirectional influence of the media on the public, suppressing the role of media in *reflecting* public opinion, accepting without question an active role for the media's creators and a passive role for everyone else.

Existing research on how the media works presents a more complex picture. A substantial part of this research is given to how reality is being 'edited', or reconstructed, in the process of becoming a media message. This process includes decisions such as what to focus on within a story, which adjectives, images, camera angles, pages or columns to use, when during the day will it be seen/heard, will there be a voice-over or a presenter, should there be pre-publicity, should it be presented as news, a documentary or fiction?

The large number of variables to be taken into account illustrates not only the choices that confront the editors, but also the components that influence the impact of the finished product. Yet perhaps the most telling element is that most of these decisions are either taken in advance (for example, for which programme the item is being prepared) or made as if intuitively, in the sense of not being premeditated, but coming out of the director's personal preferences and background.

The unidirectional perspective, of which the audience is assumed to be a recipient, does not stand up to scrutiny. The audience has the power to move from one channel to another, from one newspaper to another, to select what to read, listen to and view, and ultimately to switch off the television or not read any newspapers. In addition, each person brings her or his own set of beliefs, experiences and criteria for judging the value of a new programme/article. It is within this extremely varied background and foreground that the media works, needs to win everyday afresh, while simultaneously and relentlessly attempting to shape it.

Matters are further complicated by the specific issues that coverage of mental distress brings to the fore. The discomfort, the sense of the unknown, the unintelligible, the suffering, the failure, the shame and the guilt, the sense of threat and fear of assumed violence, the attraction of making sense of the unchartered space of the irrational and of being in touch with hidden parts of ourselves, the meeting point between science and art: all are embedded in the message of what mental distress is about. How to make sense of this bewildering array is the main issue for the media, with the specific focus shifting in accordance with a story's newsworthiness.

All of this makes it imperative to have a useful conceptual framework within which to develop a suitable methodology to study the ways in which mental distress has been treated by the media. Following a discussion of such a framework, this chapter will focus on what can be learned from the media's treatment of mental distress, based on evidence gleaned primarily during my own research on British newspapers and some television documentary programmes, and research on ten years of documentary programmes on mental distress on Italian television.

Conceptual approaches and their methodological implications

Positivist content analysis

Studies in this mould tend to perceive the media as reflecting public views, and focus on a statistical content analysis of categories such as the portrayal of people with mental illness, views on different categories of mental illness, interventions and professions. While paying attention to location in newspapers, less attention is paid to style of presentation. An underlying assumption in these studies is that decisions on content categories and coding are unproblematic provided there is interrater reliability.

Psychiatry is thus perceived as an unproblematic area of professional activity, where the views of professionals are not only correct, but should be emulated by the public.[1] Therefore when Winnick found in 1982 that public views as presented in the media had become more similar to those of the professionals than they were in the 1960s, he interpreted the findings as a sign of greater tolerance and lack of stigma. He was also reassured by the fact that most of the programmes focusing on mental illness were prepared in consultation with professionals. An unambiguous positivist, structural–functionalist, social psychological perspective is adopted.

Gerbner[2] offered a more complex analysis in suggesting that the media influences the public by cultivating a symbolic universe, which in the case of violence would lead television viewers, especially those who view it a lot, to assume that the world around them is imbued with violence. He found that people with mental illness were not only seen as violent, but also as evil. However replications of his study failed to substantiate his conceptualisation. A recent survey of two thousand people in Malvern and Bromsgrove (mid-England), where vignettes were the main research tool, has illustrated the following:[3]

- Residents of Bromsgrove seemed slightly more tolerant than those in Malvern. The authors attribute this difference to the existence of a traditional psychiatric hospital in Bromsgrove and a community-based service in Malvern.
- Tolerance was closely correlated with being younger, better educated and having personal knowledge of someone who suffers from mental illness.
- A low level of identification with sufferers was exhibited.
- A low level of knowledge of the services was demonstrated, but the residents of Malvern (which has community-based services) proposed a more enterprising approach to the use of services.

While this type of analysis whets our appetite for more information, adds little to our understanding of people's attitudes towards sufferers or the motives underlying these attitudes.

A more interactive variation of this approach is provided by Cumberbatch and Howitt,[4] who studied the active part played by both the media and the audience. They concluded that we do not have a clear idea as to how the media affects the audience, and cannot assume a clear line of influence.

This tradition is not concerned with issues such as the origins of images and attitudes, why they change when they do, and how are they related to wider issues. There is also an assumption that media expression should be taken at face value: namely that there are few contradictions to be explored, or different levels of the message. Interestingly, although the *form* aspect of the media is mentioned, this is studied only at a superficial level, such as whether a programme was factual or fictional in origin. The impact of the audiovisual effects used in a programme is left out in favour of concentrating on the content.

When images of people suffering from mental distress have been looked at in these studies, it has been found that the connotations attached to them are those of assumed criminality[5] in comparison either with people suffering from other disabilities or with people without disabilities.

The social representation approach

Within the social representation and attribution approach[6] it is assumed that we construct the meaning of our views of the world, and of ourselves, through a series of social representations. These are the product of cognitive, social and psychological stimuli processed into patterns which then structure our world view and how we continue to establish social representations. The approach attempts to combine individual with collective representations, the symbolic with the material world, and consequently is more influenced by sociology than other strands of social psychology.

The media provides a rich source of such representations. While employing an array of methodologies ranging from social psychology to structuralist anthropology, it is difficult to ascertain what constitutes a valid methodology and valid evidence for an argument put forward by a researcher. Only a few clues are offered as to why specific choices are made. For example the wish to belong to a group implies a preference for the images of oneself and one's group that are the least stigmatising, while people seen as being different are lumped together with the more negative stereotypes.

Jodelet,[7] in the study of a French 'family colony' for people with mental distress and learning difficulties described in Chapter 5, has systematically followed the social representation approach. Her study illustrates the potential richness of the approach in terms of combining different conceptual frameworks and methods. Yet without a qualm she postulates on the first page that these people are 'the other' for those with whom they live and for all outsiders. At no point is it considered that the category of 'the other' encapsulates more than one type of 'otherness', and that therefore the categorisation is too crude to tell us much about the specificity of the images of mental illness and the people who are seen as bearing it.

In a direct application of social representation to the study of the media and mental distress, Adlam[8] looked at TV news coverage of mental illness, assuming that the media shapes our social representations of mental illness by a stereotypical representation, in which people with mental illness are 'the other' in the sense of being 'absolutely different from the rest of us, either in terms of violence and crime, or in terms of being objects of pity.

Both the social psychological approach outlined above and the Marxist-discourse approach to be described below, rely to an extent on the social representation frame of reference.

The deviancy school approach

Sociological approaches to deviancy underlie – either explicitly or implicitly – the social psychological approaches mentioned above, in providing a more general framework as to why and how we as a society castigate certain groups as deviant, and the social treatment accorded to them.

Cohen[9] proposed that societies periodically go into states of 'moral panic', where a threat to core values is perceived as coming out of the actions and attitudes of a group of people. The threat, and the reactions to it, are then stylized and stereotyped by the media in headlines such as the following:

- 'Freed to kill in the community' (*Daily Express*, 2 July 1993)
- 'Cut down in a frenzy: more targets of a terrifying syndrome' (*Daily Express*, 2 July 1993)

- '33 patients who were freed to kill' (*Daily Express*, 17 August 1994)
- 'Danger on our streets' (*Tonight*, 27 September 1994)

It is tempting to propose, as Hally does,[10] that the seriously mentally ill have become the 'folk devils' of the 1990s, namely those who represent the new threat to our well-being, including our very physical existence. However Cohen's framework does not advance us much beyond stating that societies move from one set of threats with its accompanying scapegoats, to another. More specifically, his approach does not help us to understand, for example, why this is the case in Britain but not in other European countries, including Italy, where more psychiatric hospitals have been closed than in Britain.

The Marxist-discourse approach

Researchers interested in the portrayal of deviancy by the media and influenced by Marxist sociology and the analysis of literary texts have focused on exploring issues of social control, class, legitimation and ideology. Following the Marxist methodological tradition, they have investigated the dialectics development of media representation in terms of how ideological hegemony is established over time, its contradictions, and materialist and idealist levels. Their interest in the symbolic has earned them the reputation being revisionists within the Marxist camp.

By the beginning of the 1980s the discourse approach had been added to the Marxist influence, imported from Europe, through structuralism and semiotics. Deconstruction and postmodernism are also echoed at times in the writings of this loose grouping. Discourse is defined as 'both a topic and a coded set of signs through which that topic is organised, understood and made expressible, including the social process by which sense is made and reproduced'.[11]

There is a lot of interest in what is labelled 'popular', defined as rendering material familiar or acceptable to the audience, as it is argued that television is not an elitist instrument of communication, unlike newspapers. Television is seen as the confirmation of secular morality in which scientists and doctors are the heroes. This approach is interested in heroes and villains, in 'unworthy discourse' about what is labelled 'dirty', the focus on 'the community' in television, where the community is either the 'asylum of the unfit' or is recreated in the 'workplace family' as a substitute for the non-exciting or unsatisfactory real family and community. Thus television is a creation of a 'super-reality', which is less a reflection of ordinary reality and more in the business of constructing new symbolic realities.

Two specific terms are worthy of being singled out for the study of the media and mental distress. 'Dirt' is defined as the lack of boundaries, as the coexistence of ambiguities, both at the social and at the individual level.[12] A 'scandalous category' is defined as a category with a high level of dirt, containing a large number of contradictions and ambiguities, scandalising the wish for certainty, clarity and peace of mind.[13] It seems to me that mental distress is a scandalous category *par excellance*, shrouded in 'dirt' from beginning to end.

Within the approach attention is paid to style as much as to content, and to the location of items. Style includes audiovisual elements, editing and pacing. There are no clear-cut rules as to how far to go in the analysis of either the content or the form, how to construct a framework that is replicable, or how far simply to let one's poetic imagination run riot. As a *methodology in practice* it resembles literary criticism rather than a positivist piece of research, yet it is also quite unlike classical texts of semiotics.

These writers approach the media as a myth-creating instrument, in which reality is always arranged. Therefore, even in an attempt to present 'facts', the interpretative aspect comes through the mode of presentation, the selection of what to present, how much space to give to which set of facts or views, how much authority to invest in the programme (for example, whether to engage a famous presenter or employ a famous person to do the voiceover, decisions as to the amount and type of line-up given to the programme). They are interested in the *formal* message – that is the message the programme producers claim to present (the coded message) versus the *underlying* message, as interpreted by the researcher or the viewer (the decoded message). This is partly due to the assumption that in a myth we will always have more than one level of awareness and attention, and more than one type of message, but also because of the assumed inherent ambiguity of most topics and myths. Another means of unravelling the ambiguity is through *pairing* – looking at complementary and contradictory images that attempt to portray the same component, person or message.

They are also interested in categories that have been nominated explicitly versus related categories that have not been nominated, because they are taken for granted. Alternatively the ex-nominated categories have remained 'missing issues', namely related issues that are so uncomfortable to tackle that they are better left unmentioned.

Post-modernity stands for absolute relativism, for a fragmented world view.[14] In such a world people with mental illness should be less out of place, as they express absolute subjectivity and focus on emotions, two characteristics that are supposed to be the hallmark of post-modernity. At the same time, in a world so patently lacking in certainties many people look for certainties in the form of stereotypes or 'bogy people' to differentiate themselves from and to blame. This is expressed, for example, in the rampant nationalism of a variety of ethnic and cultural groups today. If this is the case, then people with mental illness will provide a ready-made case for intensifying the stereotypical approach already in existence towards them, rather than weakening this tendency.

A further implication of post-modernity is that the impact of the media is further fragmented by the audience's own framework, and depends more on momentary moods and situational reactions than on a generalised attitude.

To summarise, existing conceptual and methodological frameworks are often too simplistic and narrow in focus, or so wide-ranging as to seem confused and unsystematic. At the same time they offer a number of interesting dimensions for the study of the media and mental distress.

Methodologically, the frameworks outlined above fail to take on board the inability of the researcher *not* to have her or his own position on mental distress and how this position influences the analysis of media material. The researcher's point of view of what mental illness signifies to the media and to the public is central to the type of research to be conducted, and the ease of doing so. Those who assume that it is just a disease, or that this is how the public views it, have an easier task than those who assume that it is about ambiguity, about breaking codes of behaviour, thought, affect, disorder of a type that is not easily made sense of, which is the position of this author. Such a perspective evokes Goffman's and Scheff's assumption that mental illness is about residual rule-breaking.[15] If we accept this assumption, then the media should be analysed in terms of how it reflects such views and the meanings it attaches to mental illness.

Making sense would also need to be broken down, by using sequencing, locating specific meanings in time, space, culture, types of explanations, to mention some of the possible ways of analysis. Essentially there is no escape from having to give mental illness an *a priori* meaning in order to render the uncontrollable controllable, not in the sense of coercion, but in the sense of understanding it within one's world view. It seems to me that the Marxist-discourse tradition offers the more comprehensive conceptual and methodological framework for the study of the media and mental distress.

A second major methodological problem is how to operationalise all of what has been assumed. Appendix 7.1 summarises the content and form categories that were used in my study of newspaper articles on mental distress. The range of issues involved in the study of the interface between the media and mental distress and ways of handling them will be illustrated by examining media coverage of:

- a particularly problematic category;
- a one-off traumatic event;
- the portrayal of a major policy change over a ten-year period.

The following three examples illustrate the analytical framework discussed above.

'The tragedy of schizophrenia': an exercise in constructing new victims, heroes and villains

In December 1985 Ms M. Wallace published a series of three articles in *The Times* under the general heading 'The tragedy of schizophrenia', for which she was awarded the title 'the best investigative journalist of the year'.

The titles were:

'When freedom is a life sentence'
'A patient's cry – can nobody help?'
'No patience with former patients?'

In addition to these highly charged titles a large picture of a cross in a graveyard accompanied the second article in the series. Since then she has established an organisation called SANE (Schizophrenia A National Emergency). This organisation has been at the forefront of calling for an end to the closure of psychiatric hospitals and for the introduction of community supervision orders, as already mentioned in Chapters 2 and 4. The organisation has been successful in attracting funding and media attention, and now runs a telephone helpline that is publicised widely in London.

As the above image demonstrates, the images used by Ms Wallace are highly emotive. The language used is emotive and evocative too: 'I have never seen a human being in such an appalling state', 'its like a continual bereavement . . . the loss of your son's potential, the pain he goes through and the way people lose interest when he does not get better'. 'At 28 David is a pathetic figure, his body twitching and shaking'.

I am all for the use of emotive language when describing what mental distress is like, as it is an emotional and personal issue (as well as a scientific, social and political issue). However Ms Wallace distorts the picture considerably by neglecting the following:

1. While she states that a third of people suffering from Schizophrenia recover in full and another third recover partially, she has not interviewed even one of those who have recovered, or their relatives.
2. She states clearly that the relatives of sufferers are unsung heroes, but she does not seem even to consider that sufferers too are frontline heroes.
3. Professionals, especially social workers, are depicted as the villains of the piece, who give laughable advice to sufferers and their relatives. She is insinuating that, as in child abuse cases, social workers are responsible for the death of people suffering from mental illness or murders committed by them. Yet Ms Wallace does not provide evidence to substantiate this allegation.

4. While stating that scientific research has demonstrated the biochemical aetiology of schizophrenia, she 'forgets' to mention studies evaluating the rehabilitation of people with schizophrenia in the community in the United States Britain and Italy.

That this series of articles received an award for investigative journalism tells us something important about journalists, about the centrality of emotional hype and the readiness to turn a blind eye to major distortions by the people who manufacture news and media coverage.

The Hungerford massacre: a scandal lumped within a scandalous category

On 19 August 1987 a man shot fourteen people in the market town of Hungerford in the south of Britain before killing himself. The second person to be killed was his mother; all others seem to have been chosen at random. This was the first mass killing by one person in British history.

My interest in studying the reactions to this event arose out of seeing the headline 'Matricide points to schizophrenia' on the front page of a respected quality daily newspaper.[16] Initially I felt revulsion, and hoped that this was not a repetition of the user and professional bashing line taken in another quality paper at the end of 1986. I then thought through the likely effect of such a headline on the readers on the one hand, and the issues that the Hungerford Massacre (as it became known) would raise for newspaper editors and journalists. The following analysis is a construction of my understanding of the perspective of the latter two groups.

A study of the coverage of the event during the first week and one day a week later for rechecking purposes in four quality papers was undertaken (the *Daily Telegraph*, the *Guardian*, the *Independent* and *The Times*). These papers represent the political right through to the liberal left of centre in Britain. All columns were read to check on location and whether the location changed as the event faded, as well as for style and content. The event raised the following issues for the newspapers:

1. Giving meaning to this unexpected, and unprecedented, act of violence (contextualising and explaining, reducing the level of 'dirt').

A Scandalous Category

2. Attributing responsibility and blame.
3. Demonstrating solidarity with the bereft community.
4. Contemplating the preferred policy solutions.

Due to lack of space, only the first two issues will be looked at in this text.

This list of issues is based on the assumption that the quality papers in particular wish to be opinion leaders, and not merely reflect the news, while the event was truly sensational, these newspapers would not have wished to remain only at the level of sensational reportage. Furthermore the lifespan of interest in this event – probably no more than one week – would have had implications for the speed with which the interpretations and solutions were offered.

As a first-ever event of this kind, no straightforward interpretations and no simple solutions were available to the quality newspapers. Therefore how to handle a news item that raised many uneasy issues would have been an important issue for them. Of necessity the reportage was a reconstruction, due to the absence of the key figure, and as such was about myth creation. However even if the key figure had been available he would have been able to furnish only one perspective; as would the other participants, who took part only in some aspects of the event.

Meaning was given through the sequencing of what happened, where, when and to whom; descriptions of the main actors, of the town; a reconstruction of the history of the killer; and from there to explanations. These steps were taken simultaneously.

Contextualisation consisted mainly of describing the town on the one hand and the reconstructed life story of the killer on the other. The sense of contrast could not have been greater. Hungerford has been portrayed as the idyll of the English countryside, a leafy, sleepy, market town where a harmonious community lives. Ryan (the gunman) was described as 'a loner living in a fantasy world of violence' (*The Telegraph*, 21 August 1987). To obtain such a clear-cut contrast several 'dirt' features had to be ignored, such as variations in life-style within Hungerford depending on income and class, and whether Ryan had fit into the town in the twenty-odd years prior to the event of August 1987. Thus contextualisation left too many questions unanswered, and hence the need for an explanation.

Explanation: providing an explanation was a difficult task, given that the killing appeared to have happened totally out of the blue; that the gunman had shot himself at the end and was not available for questioning, that no motive was apparent and he had no known history of violence or mental illness. Several editorials stated the impossibility of offering an explanation, yet all of the newspapers kept attempting to come up with one. Explanations were located at two levels: Ryan's personality and life history, and general factors that might have influenced him to act in that way.

Neighbours, teachers, members of the gun club to which Ryan belonged, and later some relatives, were all approached to inform us what he was really like. In piecing this information together external contradictions were positioned as clues to internal contradictions: 'Although unemployed, he had a new car'. 'Although his mother doted on him he used to beat her up'. 'His mother was forced to work as a waitress and not only as a dinner lady in order to finance his extravagant life style'. 'He received £1000 per month left to him by his rich grandmother' (*The Times*, 22 August 1987).

It was at this stage that his past was being reconstructed. We were told of how frightened children in the area were of his driving, that he had shot cows at the age of twelve, that he had recently threatened a neighbour with a gun, and of how upset he had been at his father's funeral two years previously. The reconstruction was directly influenced by the killings, but also by the effect of the military-like suit he was wearing during the shooting and the survival kit found in the boot of his car. The possibility of him being simply evil was considered in sermons the following Sunday in the three churches of Hungerford, and was also favoured by the then prime minister, Margaret Thatcher. Such an explanation was necessary for believers to be reconvinced that God allows both evil and good to coexist, and that the choice between these two is ours alone.

However, to judge from the continuous focus in the newspapers, the location of the explanation in either evil or individual choice remained unconvincing. The newspapers then turned to experts in their attempts to provide an explanation. With one exception, all the experts were psychiatrists. The exception, a psychologist, refused to provide a diagnosis. The others suggested that he had been schizophrenic, or paranoid, or a psychopath, and might also have suffered from a brain tumour. Although most of the basic ground rules for the provision of a diagnosis could not be followed (such as seeing the patient, talking to him, to his relatives, obtaining a life and medical history), most experts were ready to go ahead and offer a label.

The most striking example of this kind was provided by a Dr Higgins, who was quoted on the front page of the *Independent* on 20 August 1987 as proposing that matricide is 'the' schizophrenic crime. No statistical proof was provided, and no textbook was mentioned. The refusal of one unnamed psychiatrist to provide a diagnosis appeared at the end of a long article, indicating its assumed insignificance.

By attaching a psychiatric diagnosis the public was being told that such behaviour can happen only when people go out of their mind. This is consoling, since the number of patently crazy people in our midst is small. Yet the 'dirt' remains, as it is all the more frightening because of the difficulty in predicting who is going to behave in this way. Several steps were taken to counter this fear. Firstly, some of the experts attempted to outline the process by which a person may come to kill *en masse*. Then other qualities of such a person were outlined. However, as some of these qualities are common to a number of people and therefore do not offer the instant ability of distinguishing a potential mass killer from the rest us (such as being a loner), ambiguity continued to reign. It was at this point that external factors were marshalled to rescue the explanatory bid. These included the easy availability of guns and ammunition and the impact of violence on television (and to a much smaller extent in films, but not in theatres and newspapers).

The ideological preferences of each newspaper come especially to the fore at that stage. For example the *Guardian* did not welcome the assertion that the massacre was a reflection of a too permissive society. The *Times* expressed an affinity with non-violent gun owners. The *Independent* was not keen on an increase in state control over the media. The *Daily Telegraph* asserted that the number of weapons found in Britain was more suited to Beirut, where presumably conflict-free communities did not exist, unlike its portrayal of Hungerford.

Reflecting the views of the readers: this was carried out overtly in the letters to the editor, and in the views expressed in editorials.

Both were subject to selection by the editors. Nearly all of the letters were about gun laws, and nearly all were from men (whereas most of the victims were women). A minority of the letters were concerned with violence in the media and the suitability of increasing state control over the media as a solution. Only three letters pointed out that people diagnosed as suffering from schizophrenia are as unlikely to kill their mothers as the rest of us.

Two unintended results came to the fore as a result of the media coverage of this event: provision of a powerful motive for an increase in state control over the media, and intensification of the myth of violence as an integral part of serious mental distress.

The newspapers provided information, but also acted as gatekeepers to information and views. They were confronted with an impossible task, which was largely off-loaded into the scandalous category, and one major function of this category is to provide a solution to the impossible.

Reflecting on and reacting to a major policy shift: ten years of newspaper and documentary television coverage of the italian psychiatric reform, 1978–88

The Italian psychiatric reform provides an interesting case for studying the interface between the media and mental distress. It had a number of dramatic features that the media found difficult to resist. These included the closure of hospitals and the celebrations that went with them, as well as the passing a national law following a national referendum, and it continues to upset many people such as professionals, informal carers and relatives, and some middle-class people suffering from nimby ('not in *my* back yard') effect.

The initiators of the reform openly courted local and national media people to establish public support so as to compensate for the lack of support from the majority of professionals and politicians. Their successors have continued this tradition. Moreover some of the reformers are in the business of encouraging the production of culture as a tool of both production and attitudinal change (see Chapter 6).[17] A number of studies of newspapers' reactions have been carried out by Italian researchers. Most of them focus on comparing one or two national papers at two points in time, usually at the beginning of the national reform

(1978) and a few years later (1983). These predominantly follow the traditional content analysis approach, in which it is assumed that it is unproblematic to investigate the media effect and/or mental illness as reflected in the media.

Content-wise the newspapers demonstrate more interest in mental illness than is the case in the United State and Britain and on the whole a more positive attitude towards people with mental illness, although more positive at the beginning of the national psychiatric reform (the early 1980s) than towards the end of the 1980s. While no wish to reopen the hospitals was expressed, this was accompanied by a wish not to be closely associated with people suffering from mental illness. Italian researchers also looked at the newspapers' view of the psychiatric services and came up with a rather lukewarm, if not straightforwardly negative, overall opinion of their performance.[18]

Italian television documentary programmes on mental distress, 1978–88
The following analysis is based on fifteen hours of documentary programmes and two hours of news bulletins. While not a representative sample of all of that was produced in Italy during this period, the seventeen hours provide enough of the flavour of the way the Italian psychiatric reform was portrayed by the television network.

Methodologically, the material was analysed according to the following categories: main content (the portrayal of and views on service users, mental illness, mental health, relatives, services and professionals, policy); global message (looking for levels of messages, contradictions, complementarity, nominated and ex-nominated categories); and style variables and their effect on the content. An Italian colleague, Monica Savio, a sociologist who researched the development of community psychiatric nursing in Britain and Italy, has also independently rated the material as a check on the reliability and validity of my own rating.

In general, documentary programmes started with a 'starry-eyed' approach towards the reform in 1978. While this offered a propaganda coup to the initiators of the reform, it did not result in interesting programmes, either artistically, intellectually or emotionally. People with mental distress were portrayed primarily as dim victims of social circumstances and inexplicable cruelty, with some flashes of originality.

For example M., a young man who had spent many years in hospital was filmed at the hospital when it became an open institution. Filmed against the background of the hospital's splendid gardens, he spoke about the loss of his civil rights and the importance of regaining these rights, about himself as an original poet and thinker, but one without money and therefore an object of ridicule. All the time his leg was moving uncontrollably. The carrier of a scandalous category is on the one hand portrayed as any other young man with ambitions and lack of resources, and on the other hand as someone with unrealistic expectations of life and retribution, and an unexplainable past.

Subsequent programmes from the mid-1980s focused on much a narrower canvas, such as the past of a client and a critical incident in her life at present as a way of illustrating how a service works. This had greater emotional resonance and enabled the viewer to stay longer with the story, while taking on board the activities of the service and its philosophy as background information. From the mid-1980s onward critical views of the reform were expressed too, mainly by relatives, but also by professionals and a few politicians. The criticisms pertained more to what was not being offered in supporting relatives and providing asylum facilities, than to a rejection of the reform.

A tearful, desperate mother phoned in during a programme on an ex-patients' work cooperative in Turin. The viewers could not see her, but she was clearly audible. What she had to say was not censored, and it was difficult to interrupt her flow. The presenter seemed to be on the verge of losing control of the programme. The woman did not live in the Turin area, and there was very little that could be offered to her on the spot. She was listened to with respect and growing sympathy, and some of the members of the cooperative suggested that her son could join them as a solution to her – and his – problem. Stylistically the programme combined a panel discussion, with the audience chipping in, and a phone-in section.

Another programme covered a public meeting on the reform. Relatives for and against the reform quarrelled openly and bitterly, while some of the professionals present attempted unsuccessfully to gain control. This programme was shot in Arezzo, a well-off town in Tuscany. Its place in the history of the Italian reform is due to group of the founders of the psychiatric reform that led to the closure of the local mental hospital at the beginning of the 1980s and to the restructuring of the mental health services. A second programme, filmed in the same area, was one of the few portrayals on Italian television of threatened violence by a service user. First a middle-class woman, a local magistrate, described how threatening she found this man, that he had hurled stones on the street and looked menacing. The camera then showed the man playing with an iron rod on fire in a blackened room that seemed to be a blacksmith's workshop. He looked strange and said little. His father – with whom he lived – and the service workers who were interviewed also acknowledged that he could be violent, but only if provoked. This was juxtaposed with an interview of the extended family of another ex-resident of the psychiatric hospital, who were much happier about him living outside the hospital, near them but not with them. Reflecting this happier state, they were interviewed under a wide, majestic tree. The overall impression is of television footage accompanying a process in the making, rather than expressing a judgement.

While more critical comments were made about the reform in the late 1980s, respect towards the reformers and a growing respect towards service users were in evidence. Extremely little was mentioned either about mental illness or classical forms of intervention, be they drugs or psychotherapy. Was a new myth being created, in which the social, cultural, political and subjective suffering were the foreground issues, bringing with them different types of 'dirt'?

The richness of the material, in terms of both stimuli and interpretation possibilities, is well illustrated by ten minutes of a popular chat show (the Maurizio Costanzo Show) with a live audience in a well-known theatre hall in Rome. Filmed in March 1990 it contained three items on mental illness and health, two related to each other, and three protagonists: a politician, a writer and an ex-resident of a psychiatric hospital, who lived there for forty years before resettling outside. Thus matters relating to mental distress have become part of the production of culture (literature and politics) and entertainment (popular culture).

The politician was a 40-year-old male MP for the Radical Party, a small, liberal, humanist party that had traditionally campaigned for human rights. He had been asked to the programme to tell the tale of the exposure of a recent scandal in a psychiatric and learning difficulties hospital in Agrigento, a medium-sized town in Sicily.

The scandal, which he had helped to expose via newspapers, television and the Italian parliament, focused on the horrendous living conditions of the residents in that institution. They were neither fed nor clad properly, sanitation was beyond the pale, and the money earmarked for the place went to the local Mafia branch. The whistle had been blown by workers, who had endangered their lives by pointing their fingers at the Mafia protégés who were running the institution. The MP followed the exposure not only by insisting on an enquiry, an immediate improvement of the physical conditions of the institution and the removal of the director, but also by organising a solidarity concert on the hospital grounds, at which the residents – now well fed and well dressed – were the guests of honour and to which nationally famous artists contributed free of charge.

During the programme the MP went on to say how surprised he had been by the ability of the residents, especially the women among them, to enjoy the concert. Contrasting shots of the institution and its residents during the pre-exposure and post-exposure periods of the scandal provided the background for his interview on the chat show.

This an interesting example of how entertainment can be used to express solidarity, how the media can contribute positively by both reflecting and shaping public opinion. Even more intriguing was the process by which patients who initially resembled animals, evoking pity and disgust, became endowed with a major positive human quality, namely the ability to enjoy themselves in a dignified way.

The amount of 'dirt' in this cameo was very high. Indignation was projected at the director of the institute and the Mafia, a rather powerful – if hated – group. No doubt was expressed as to whether the residents, an unproductive element of the town's society, deserved better; and the issue of their assumed illness and disability faded into the background, while issues of poverty and misery came to the fore. The residents were judged instinctively as worthy of demonstrable solidarity, not only by the MP and the artists, but also by the producer/presenter of the show. By inviting the MP to reconstruct the story he demonstrated that the story was newsworthy and of entertainment value.

The MP's discourse was followed by an exchange between the presenter and an attractive, giggly, 'sexy' woman promoting the virtues of a chat show on a mattress, because, according to her, this was the only place where people could really relax. Observing the non-verbal communications of other members of the panel it was easy to spot that a woman on the right-hand side of the stage found this exchange distasteful. She was Chiara Sasso, a writer of novels who had spent two years with the residents of a hospital that was in the process of closing: she wrote a poetic book about the experience, ironically entitled 'Ten Thousand Sheets Later'. When the presenter questioned her about her reasons for being there and writing the book, she seemed to look for a way of not answering the question herself, and suggested that Rosanna – an ex-resident sitting in the audience – be asked to contribute.

Thus the main 'mental health star' of that show was ushered in: Rosanna, a tall woman of 58 with a 'lived-in' face, few teeth and a huge, warm smile. She spoke about coming to Rome for the first time for the show, marvelling at the sights, her admiration for the presenter, her identification with Giulietta Messina, the waif prostitute in a film by Fellini, about being rescued from beating and hunger by becoming mad and being in hospital, and about being rescued again by being encouraged to leave the hospital and live in the community. She and Chiara Sasso talked about seeing her home for the first time in 40 years – at night, as she was afraid of being rejected again – and of the love–hate relationship she had with the town.

A sense of awe was felt at the lady who had been hospitalised for so long, yet used language in a poetic way and seemed sophisticated, cultured, curious about life and able to enjoy it much more than most ordinary people. A sense of amazement emanated from the presenter – sweating, visibly touched by her, yet wanting to stop her so that the show could continue as planned, but at the same time not daring to do so.

From this example it seems that within twenty years Italian society has moved from total rejection of people within that scandalous category of mental distress to them becoming active creators of mass culture. Of course one swallow does not mean that spring has arrived, and I am not attempting to argue that all people with mental distress have become valued producers of culture in Italy. But Maurizio Costanzo's decision that not only an MP who had exposed a mental health scandal, but also a writer on a psychiatric hospital and an ex-resident were of good entertainment value without the need to make fun of them is in itself a reflection of that sea change. That they were put together with the sexy starlet and other celebrities of dubious reputation is perhaps an illustration of the post-modern world in which we live.

The postscript to the programme introduced yet another twist to the complex reality with which the programme was attempting to come to terms. After the programme Rosanna had many admiring letters. However Maurizio Constanzo received threatening phone calls from professionals insinuating unprofessional conduct by him and accusing him of exploiting Rosanna for commercial purposes. A promised sequel with Rosanna was therefore abandoned, even though she was flown once more to Rome and lavishly entertained by the presenter.

Rosanna finally received her promised sequel in 1992, a one-hour programme focused entirely on her – on the main public television channel, but at midnight. Rosanna recalled her pre-hospital, hospital and post-hospital life, adopting an unflattering stance towards herself and others, and laying the main blame on structural deprivation. Her humanity, sense of humour and intelligence shone throughout this programme, together with a sense of toughness that I had not observed in the previous show. Artistically this was a difficult programme to make, as there was only one protagonist. The producer and director made much play of her face, using different lightening angles, but curiously did not invite other people to speak or make her move from her chair.

I have been told that Rosanna is now a media star and that she has used the media successfully to prevent the removal of the many cats she looks after at the group home she shares with other ex-patients. It can be safely presumed that the support workers and the other residents are less than happy about Rosanna's rise as a media star.

Concluding comments

The examples described in this chapter have covered the extremes and only a fraction of the vast range of the arena of mental distress.

In 'The tragedy of schizophrenia' a most selective picture was provided, aimed at creating a specific emotional atmosphere, with scant regard for facts and alternative perspectives.

In the Hungerford Massacre coverage, mental distress was used as a way of preventing debate on the issues that that tragic event had raised. In this way the level of 'dirt' was disguised and a scandalous category was employed to bring the tragedy – for which there were no easy or simple solutions – to a close. The stereotyping of people diagnosed as suffering from schizophrenia has increased, at least in the coverage of the quality papers, which is another means of decreasing the level of ambiguity. Yet interestingly enough the reactions of the readers have not focused on mental illness, but on violence in its relationship to gun ownership and to television. It would seem that this implies that the stereotyping was taken for granted and therefore not even worth bothering about, as in the debate on violence it is assumed that the risk of another mass killing relates to other mentally ill people having access to guns or being influenced by violence on the screen.

Insinuation, rather than evidence, was used throughout by the newspapers in arguing the case that Ryan must have been mad. If quality newspapers consider this level of misinformation as adequate and responsible coverage, it is unlikely that attitudes among the educated middle classes towards people with serious mental distress will become more open-ended and more open to seeking out and taking on board proper information.

The coverage on Italian television has been more wide-ranging and more open-ended. In the programme looked at above – the Maurizio Constanzo show – the audience was told very little about mental illness itself, but was told quite a lot about the people suffering from it, both as people and as objects of neglect and stigmatisation. The audience was also given a mixed, very 'dirty' message about the workers in the mental health services. On the one hand they were portrayed as rescuers and benefactors. On the other hand they were the cynical exploiters of defenceless people.

The issue of the potential, or actual, violence of people with serious mental distress did not come up in most of the Italian programmes. This must have been a conscious decision on the part of the producers and directors of these programmes, as it is always possible to find a person who has acted violently and strangely.

To the extent that there is a direct relationship between the unfolding of psychiatric reform in Italy and the way mental distress is portrayed, then the reform has led to a less stigmatising approach and to a greater readiness to look at people who embody it as people first and objects second. The 'scandal' value turns from the threatening element in the connotation of the 'scandalous' to that of curiosity and entertainment value.

Both the British and the Italian examples treated the key protagonist as 'the other'. However the meaning attached to that otherness differs considerably. In the case of Ryan, 'the other' is portrayed as menacing and murderous due to mental illness. In the case of Rosanna, 'the other' is someone who has managed to retain her humanity despite years of deprivation and oppression.

Even in those few British television programmes in which people with mental distress have appeared, they have not been encouraged to tell their tale in a way that would have revealed much about them as people, rather than as sufferers of mental distress. Can it be argued that the greater openness demonstrated on Italian television towards people with mental distress and towards the category itself is due to the impact of the psychiatric reform? Or was it that the reform became possible because Italians were more open in their approach than the British public was/is?

Not having the baseline information on attitudes in the 1960s and early 1970s in Italy, it is not possible to provide definitive answers to these questions. But the large number of social reforms undertaken in the early 1970s in Italy would indicate a greater public readiness to adopt a more open-ended approach to mental distress too, starting with a belief in the relationship between social deprivation and mental distress, rather than in the pure disease model of mental illness.

In all probability the reform has enhanced this approach, without attempting to change the range of public beliefs on the causes of mental illness. The visibility of people with mental distress who individually demonstrated that they were on the whole able to live outside a total institution gave credibility to the ideals of the reform. This overall credibility has remained, even if in more than one area the reality of the services and the attitude of the public and the politicians falls short of the ideal.

If anything, the opposite has happened in Britain, despite the policy of hospital closure and resettling former residents in the community since the 1980s. While there is less fear of allowing the 'old long stay' group to resettle, belief in the disease model has increased and is reinforced by the dominant professional group and relatives. Perhaps not surprisingly this has led to a reforging of the *assumed* relationship between mental distress and criminality in relation to the 'new long stay'. This may be combined with the guilt that is felt about the visible and increasing homelessness of young people, with racism, and with fear of young men with mental distress, who are seen as more difficult to control and contain than the old long stay group.

This text cannot even attempt to answer the question of why British professionals and the British public differ from their Italian counterparts, beyond pointing out the different social contexts at crucial historical moments. All of what has been attempted here has been aimed at highlighting how these differences are reflected in the media coverage of that scandalous category *par excellance* – mental distress.

In the discussion of the proposed British legislation on community supervision orders in Chapter 4 it was mentioned that Britain rates second highest in Europe in the number of people it imprisons, while Italy rates fourth from the bottom of that list. Thus it is suggested that attitudes to law and order issues are at the core of British attitudes to people with mental illness, and that the British media reflects and further shapes such attitudes in its coverage. Much more research on these issues in other European countries is needed if we are to gain a clearer picture

The divergence from traditional approaches to mental distress observed in the Italian media, and to a lesser extent in the British media, also lend some credibility to the post-moderinist argument of shifts and more open-ended reappraisal in people's views about controversial areas, of which mental distress is one.

Appendix 7.1: schedule for the analysis of TV items on the Italian psychiatric reform

1. Content
2. Context factors
3. The level at which images are set
4. Normative behaviour
   - Patients
   - Relatives
   - The general public
5. The mental health service
6. Pressure groups
7. Policy
8. The audience
9. The discourse
10. The style
    - Tone of presentation
    - Sound elements
    - Visual style

Epilogue

> In another age, I would be a witch. I live alone with two cats. I like to spend time alone. If I need a conversation I talk to my cats and my aspidistra, Benjamin, who has been with me for 30 years. I would like always to wear sloppy comfortable clothes. I would like to spend more time alone than I do now with my activist and money-earning schedule.
>
> As women get older we get increasingly less powerful in society. I do still want to be heard on the subject of psychiatric abuse. I watch with anger the deterioration on drugs of some fellow members of survivors groups who still obey the psychiatric order to take them for life. There are still no strong alternatives to psychiatry for them to choose (Viv Lindow, *Asylum Magazine*, vol. 7, no 4, 1993, p. 7).

In 1993 Dr Viv Lindow was the chairperson of Survivors Speak Out, one of the most active service user groups in Europe.

In this book I have attempted to offer information, share experiences and provide an analysis, rather than suggest that ready-made solutions exist just around the corner. The incredible richness of thought and initiative in mental health systems that has emerged since 1980 has been outlined. At the same time the text has highlighted an incredible poverty of genuine dialogue between those who have power and those who do not, in integrating the richness into a viable and coherent lifeline for direct and indirect sufferers of mental distress. In this maze we could do with some good 'witches' to guide us. We need the humility to:

- accept how much we still do not know;
- listen much more carefully and openly to those with less power;
- have the courage to take away power from those who have too much of it;
- enable those with less power to have the ability to take power and put it to good use;
- finally accept that mental distress is not a unidimensional phenomenon;

- get rid of solutions that have proved damaging, while resourcing more promising solutions;
- invest in thinking *together* before rushing to do things separately;
- create genuine partnerships and caring to reduce suicide and murder, rather than continue the 'lock them up and stuff them with medication' approach;
- accept that Europeans have a lot to learn from – and give to – each other in the field of mental health.

Jacques Brel wrote that there are two types of time: the time that waits and the time that hopes:

> Il y a deux sortes de temps
> Ya le temps qui attend
> Et le temps qui espere.

I hope that we have reached the second type of time, and that this book will assist its readers' achievements of the objectives listed above.

References

Introduction

1. S. Mangen (ed.), *Mental Health Care in the European Community* (London: Croom Helm, 1985); H. Freeman and J. Henderson (eds), *Evaluation of Comprehensive Care of the Mentally Ill* (London: Gaskell, 1991); C. Louzon (ed.) *Sante Mentale: Realites Europeannes* (Paris: Eres, 1993).
2. M. McCrone and G. Strathdee, 'Needs not diagnosis: Towards a More Rational Approach to Community Mental Health Resourcing in Britain', *International Journal of Social Psychiatry*, vol. 40, no. 2, p. 83.
3. C. Louzoun, 'New and Old Mental Health European Realities', paper presented at the conference Recomincare di Essre, USL 24, Turin, 16 December 1993.

Prologue

1. J. K. Wing, *Reasoning about Madness* (Oxford: Oxford University Press, 19780.
2. M. Jahoda, *Current Concepts of Positive Mental Health* (New York: Basic Books, 1958).
3. S. Fernando, *Race, Culture and Mental Health* (Basingstoke: Mind Macmillan, 1991).
4. D. Jodelet, *Social Representation of Mental Illness* (Hemel Hampstead: Harvester-Wheatsheaf, 1991).
5. Mental Health Foundation, *Mental Illness: The Fundamental Facts* (London: The Mental Health Foundation, 1992).
6. S. Platt and N. Krietman, (eds), *Current Research on Suicide and Parasuicide* (Edinburgh: Edinburgh University Press, 1990).
7. R. F. W. Diekstra, R. Maris, S. Platt, A. Schmidtke and G. Sonneck (eds), *Suicide and its Prevention* (Leiden: E. J. Brill, 1989).
8. P. Crepet, G. Ferrari, S. Platt and M. Bellini (eds), *Suicidal Behaviour in Europe: Recent Research Trends* (London: John Libbey, 1992).
9. J. G. Sampio Faria, Introduction to: R. F. W. Diekstra *et al.*, op. cit., p. 9; R. F. W. Diekstra, 'Epidemiology of suicide: aspects of definition, classification and preventive policies', in R. F. W. Diekstra *et al.*, op. cit., p. 29.
10. P. Harmat, 'The Sociology of Suicide in Hungary', in S. Platt and N. Kreitman, op. cit., p. 22–9.

11. E. Durkheim, *Le Suicide* (Paris: Alcan, 1897), *Suicide: A Study in Sociology* (London: Routledge, 1952).
12. R. Sainsbury, 'The social correlates of suicide in Europe', in R. D. T. Farmer and S. K. Hirsch (eds), *The Suicide Syndrome* (London: Croom Helm, 1982).
13. R. F. W. Diekstra, 'Epidemiology of suicide', op. cit., p. 28.
14. A. P. Visser and A. J. F. M. Kerkhof, 'Suicide Attempters' attitudes towards short-term treatment on a psychiatric ward in a university hospital', in S. Platt and N. Krietman (eds) op. cit., pp. 133–45; R. Jack, *Women and Attempted Suicide* (Hove: Lawrence Erlbaum, 1992).
15. R. Jack, op. cit.
16. S. Blumenthal, V. Bell, N. U. Neumann, R. Schuttler, and R. Vogel 'Mortality and rate of suicide among first admission psychiatric patients', in S. Platt and N. Krietman, op. cit. pp. 58–66; M. Woldersdorf, P. Barth, B. Steiner, F. Keller and R. Vogel, 'Schizophrenia and suicide in psychiatric in-patients', ibid. pp. 67–77; A. Rhode, A. Marneros and A. Deister, 'Suicidal behaviour in schizophrenic patients: a follow-up investigation', ibid, pp. 78–87.
17. P. Casey, 'Parasuicide and personality disorder', in R. F. W. Diekstra *et al.*, op. cit., pp. 276–83.
18. Ibid, pp. 282.
19. S. Blumenthal *et al.*, op. cit., pp. 61.
20 R. Jack, op. cit.
21 A. T. Beck, R. A. Steer, M. Kovacs and B. Garrison 'Hopelessness and Eventual Suicide: A 10-year study of patients hospitalised with suicidal ideation', *American Journal of Psychiatry*, vol. 142 (1985), pp. 559–63.
22. R. Jack, op. cit.

1 Emerging Policy Perspectives

1. D. Robbins, *Marginalisation and social exclusion, Report to the European Commission* (Brussels: Commission of European Communities, 1990).
2. P. Spicker, *Principles of Social Welfare: An Introduction to Thinking about the Welfare State* (London: Routledge, 1988).
3. D. Piachaud and M. Kleinman, 'European Social Policy: Conceptions and Choices', *European Social Policy*, vol. 3, no. 1 (1993); P. Levin, *The Making of European Social Policy: Or, Academic concepts vs. Political Realities* (London: Department of Social Administration, London School of Economics, June 1993).
4. S. Ramon, (ed.), *Psychiatric Hospitals Closure: Myths and Realities* (London: Chapman Hall, 1992).
5. S. Ramon, *Psychiatry in Britain: Meaning and Policy* (London: Croom Helm, 1985).
6. P. Hall, H. Land, R. Parker and A. Webb, *Change, Choice and Conflict in Social Policy* (London: Heinmann, 1975).

7. J. Habermans, *Legitimation Crisis* (London: Heinmann, 1976).
8. C. Oancea, 'The Reform of Mental Health Care in Romania', paper presented at the First PRISM Conference, Community Care: Making It Work (London, Institute of Psychiatry, 13–16 November 1993.
9. L. Hantrais, *Social Policy in the European Community* (London: Macmillan, 1994).
10. G. Room, (ed.), *Anti-poverty Action-Research in Europe* (Bristol: School for Advanced Urban Studies, 1993); M.G. Giannichedda, *Italian Projects Evaluation Report* (Sassari: University of Sassari, 1989).
11. M.G. Madianos and J. Yfantopolous, *The First Monitoring Report on the Greek Psychiatric Reform: EEC Regulation 815/84* (Brussels: Commission of the European Communities DGV, 1984); C. Strutti and S. Rauber, 'Leros and the Greek mental Health System', *International Journal of Social Psychiatry*, vol. 40, no. 4 (1994); J. Yfantopoulos, 'Economic and Legal Aspects of Mental Health Policies in Greece', *International Journal of Social Psychiatry*, vol. 40, no. 4 (1994).
12. P. Warr, *Work, Unemployment and Mental Health* (Oxford: Oxford University Press, 1987). For figures on poverty in Europe see Figure 1 in G. Room (ed.), *Anti-poverty Action-research in Europe* (Bristol: SAUS, 1993), pp. 12–13. For a discussion on marginalisation see ibid, pp. 15–19 and ref. 1 above.
13. J. Le Grand and W. Bartlet (eds), *Quasi-Markets and Social Policy* (London: Macmillan, 1993).
14. T. Van der Grinten, 'Mental Health Care in the Netherlands', in S. Mangen (ed.), *Mental Health Care in the European Community* (London: Croom Helm, 1985), pp. 208–27.
15. S. Mangen (ed.), *Mental Health Care in the European Community* (London: Croom Helm, 1985).
16. M. Jones, *Social Psychiatry* (London: Tavistock, 1952); K. Jones, *The History of Mental Health Services in Britain* (London: Routledge, 1972); D. Mauri (ed.), *La Liberta e Terapeutica?* (Rome: Fletrinelli, 1986).
17. P. Chamberlayne, 'Transitions in the Private Sphere in Eastern Germany', in W. R. Lee and E. Rosenhaft (eds), *The State and Social Change in Germany 1880–1980* (Bonn: Berg, 1994); J. Finch, *Family Obligations and Social Change* (Cambridge: Polity Press, 1989); C. Ungerson, *Policy is Personal – Sex, Gender and Informal Care* (London: Tavistock, 1987); J. Lewis and B. Meredith, *Daughters who Care* (London: Routledge, 1987); J. Morris, *Independent Lives: Community Care and Disabled People* (London: Macmillan, 1993).
18. F. Basaglia, 'Problems of Law and Psychiatry: The Italian Experience', *International Journal of Law and Psychiatry*, vol. 3, (1980); pp. 17–37; L. Mosher, 'Italy's Revolutionary Mental Health Law: An Assessment', *American Journal of Psychiatry*, vol. 139, (1982), pp. 199–203.
19. J. Busfield, *Managing Madness* (London: Hutchinson, 1986); S. Goodwin, 'Community Care for the Mentally Ill in England and

Wales: myths, assumptions and realities', *Journal of Social Policy*, vol. 18, no. 1 (1989), pp. 27–52; C. Louzoun, (ed.), *Sante Mentale: Realite Europennes* (Paris: Eres, 1993); S. Mangen, (ed.), *Mental Health Care in the European Community* (London: Croom Helm, 1985); S. Ramon (ed.), *Psychiatry in Transition: British and Italian Experiences* (London: Pluto Press, 1990).

20. U. Brinck, 'Psychiatric Care and Social Support for People with Long-term Mental Illness in Sweden', *International Journal of Social Psychiatry*, vol. 40, no. 4 (1994); P. Crepet, 'A Transition Period in Psychiatric Care in Italy Ten Years after the Reform', *British Journal of Psychiatry*, vol. 156 (1990), pp. 27–36, R. Hill, 'Selected Issues in Mental Health: An Introductory Paper Prepared for the Mental Health Foundation Inquiry into Community Care for Severely Mentally Ill People (London: Research and Development in Psychiatry, November 1993); S. Mangen, 'Psychiatric Policies: Developments and Constraints', in S. Mangen (ed.), *Mental Health Care in the European Community* (London: Croom Helm, 1985), pp. 21–2; Psychosoziale Umschau: Abschluberichet der Expertenkomission zum Modellprogramm der Bundesregierung in komprimierter Form veroffentlicht (Bonn: Psychiatrieverlag, Heft 4, Dez. 1988); C. Strutti and S. Rauber, 'Leros and the Greek Mental Health System', *International Journal of Social Psychiatry*, vol. 40, no. 4 (1994); V. Svab-Cotic, 'The Continuing Care Client in Slovenia', *International Journal of Social Psychiatry*, vol. 40, no. 4 (1994).

21. I. Goffman, *Asylums* (Harmondsworth: Penguin, 1961); F. Basaglia, (ed.), *L'istuzione Negata* (Milano: Einuadi, 1968); P. Hall and I. Brockington (eds), *The Closure of Mental Hospitals* (London: Gaskell, 1990); J. Chamberlin, *On Our Own* (London: Mind Publications, 1988); M. O'Hagan, *Stopovers on My Way Home from Mars: A Winston Churchill Fellowship Report on the Psychiatric Survivor Movement in the USA, Britain and the Netherlands* (London: Survivors Speak Out, 1993).

22. L. Stein and M. A. Test (eds), *The Training in Community Living Model: A Decade of Experience*, New Directions for Mental Health Service, 26 (San Francisco: Jossey-Bass, 1985); L. Burti and L. Mosher, *Community Mental Health: Principles and Practices* (New York: Norton, 1989); T. Wainwright, 'The Changing Perspective of a Resettlement Team', in S. Ramon (ed.), *Psychiatric Hospitals Closure: Myths and Realities* (London: Chapman & Hall, 1992), pp. 43–48.

23. The British figure is cited in *The Mental Health Foundation Inquiry into Community Care for Severely Mental Ill People* (London: Mental Health Foundation, 1993); The Italian figure is cited in M. Tansella (ed.), *Community based psychiatry: long-term patterns of care in South Verona*, Psychological Medicine Monograph supplement, 19 (Cambridge: Cambridge University Press, 1991).

24. A. Scull, *Decarceration* (Englewood Cliffs, NJ: Prentice-Hall, 1978).

25. S. Mangen and F. Castel, 'France: The "Psychiatrie De Secteur" ', in S. Mangen (ed.), *Mental Health Care in the European Community* (London: Croom Helm, 1985); R. Amiel, 'France', in H. Freeman

and J. Henderson (eds), *Evaluation of Comprehensive Care of the Mentally Ill* (London: Gaskell, 1991); J. Comellos, 'The Dilemmas of Chronicity in Spain', *International Journal of Social Psychiatry*, vol. 40, no. 4 (1994); U. Brinck, 'Psychiatric Care and Social Support for People with Long-Term Mental Illness in Sweden', *International Journal of Social Psychiatry*, vol. 40, no. 4 (1994).

26. J. M. Caldas-Almeida, 'Portugal', in H. Freeman and J. Henderson (eds), *Evaluating Comprehensive Care of the Mentally Ill* (London: Gaskell, 1991).
27. M. Beeforth, E. Conlan, V. Field, B. Hoser and L. Sayce, *Whose Service Is It Anyway? Users' views on coordinating community care* (London, Research and Development in Psychiatry, The Sainsbury Centre for Mental Health, 1990).
28. D. Tomlinson, *Utopia, Community Care and the Retreat from the Asylum* (Milton Keynes: The Open University, 1991); T. Wainwright, 'The Changing Perspective of a Resettlement Team', in S. Ramon (ed.), *Psychiatric Hospital Closure* (London: Chapman & Hall, 1992), pp. 3–48.
29. K. Wright, *Cost-effectiveness in Community Care* (York: Centre for Health Economics, University of York, 1987); M. Knapp, P. Cambridge, C. Thomason, J. Beecham, C. Allen and R. Darton, *Care in the Community: Challenge and Demonstration* (Canterbury: Personal Social Services Research Unit, University of Kent, 1992).
30. M. O'Donoll, 'Cost Effectiveness of Community Care for the Chronic Mentally Ill', in H. Freeman and J. Henderson (eds), *The Evaluation of Comprehensive Care of the Mentally Ill* (London: Gaskell, 1991), pp. 174–96.
31. Knapp *et al.*, *Care in the Community*, op. cit.
32. L. M. Davies and M. F. Drummond, 'Assessments of Costs and Benefits of Drug Therapy for Treatment Resistant Schizophrenia in the United Kingdom', *British Journal of Psychiatry*, vol. 162 (1993), pp. 38–42.
33. Ibid., p. 38.
34. Mental Health Act Commission, *Fifth Biennial Report* (Nottingham: Mental Health Act Commission, HMSO, 1993); D. Pilgrim and A. Rogers, 'The Mental Health Act Commission: Four Years on', *The Psychologist's Bulletin* (Leicester: The British Psychological Society, 1988).
35. M. Barnes, R. Bowel and M. Fisher, *Sectioned: Approved Social Work and the 1983 Mental Health Act* (London: Routledge, 1990).

2 Conceptual Innovations

1. A. Lavender and F. Holloway (eds), *Community Care in Practice: Services for continuing care clients* (Chichester: Wiley, 1988).
2. M. A. Test and L. Stein (eds), *Alternatives to Mental Hospital Treatment* (New York: Plenum, 1980).

3. P. Henry, 'Towards a Rehabilitative Psychiatry', in S. Ramon (ed.), *Psychiatry in Transition* (London: Pluto, 1990), pp. 82–90.
4. L. Ciompi, 'The social outcome of schizophrenia', in J. K. Wing (ed.) *Rehabilitation of Patients with Schizophrenia and Depression* (Bern: Hans Huber, 1981).
5. A. Melluci, 'Ten Hypothees for the analysis of New Movements', in D. Pinto (ed.), *Contemporary Italian Sociology* (Cambridge: Cambridge University Press, 1981), pp. 173–94.
6. C. McCourt, Perring, 'The experience and perspectives of patients and care staff in the transition from hospital to community-based care', in S. Ramon (ed.), *Psychiatric Hospitals Closure: Myths and Realities* (London: Chapman & Hall, 1992), pp. 122–68.
7. J. Swain, V. Finkelstein, S. French, and M. Oliver (eds), *Disabling Barriers – Enabling Environments* (Milton Keyens: The Open University Press, 1993).
8. G. Breakwell, *Coping with Threatened Identities* (London: Methuen, 1986).
9. S. Ramon, 'The Relevance of Symbolic Interaction Perspectives to the Conceptual and Practice Construction of Leaving a Psychiatric Hospital', *Social Work and Social Science Review*, Summer 1990.
10. I. Goffman, 'The Moral Career of the Mentally Ill Patient', in *Asylum* (New York: Anchor, 1961).
11. J. Segal, 'The Professional Perspective', in S. Ramon (ed.), *Beyond Community Care: Normalisation and Integration Work* (London: Macmillan, 1991), pp. 85–113.
12. L. Bachrach, 'The urban environment and mental health', *International Journal of Social Psychiatry*, vol. 38, no 1 (1992), pp. 5–15; J. R. Hollingworth and E. J. Hollingworth (eds), *Care of the Chronically and Severely Ill: Comparative Social Policies* (New York: Aldine de Gruyter, 1994); R. Schulz and J. Greenlay (eds), *Innovations in Community Mental Health* (New York: Praeger, 1995).
13. J. K. Wing and R. Furlong, 'A haven for the severely disabled within the context of a comprehensive psychiatric community service', *British Journal of Psychiatry*, vol. 149 (1986), pp. 449–57.
14. R. Wykes, 'A hostel-ward for "new" long-stay patients: an evaluative study', in J. K. Wing (ed.), *Long-term Community Care: Experience in a London Borough*, Psychological Medicine Monographs, Supplement 2 (Cambridge: Cambridge University Press, 1982).
15. W. Boyde, *The Report of the Confidential Enquiry into Homicides* (London: Department of Health, HMSO, 1994); P. Crepet, 'A Transition Period in Psychiatric Care in Italy: ten years after the reform', *British Journal of Psychiatry*, vol. 156, pp. 27–38.
16. S. Cohen, *Folk Devils and Moral Panics* (Oxford: Oxford University Press, 1980).
17. SANE Posters' Campaign, London, 1989.
18. O. Gillie, 'Matricide points to Schizophrenia', *The Independent*, 20 August 1987.
19. B. Nirje, 'The Normalisaiton Principle and Its Human Management Implications', in R. Kugel and W. Wolfensberger (eds), *Changing*

Patterns in Residential Services for the Mentally Retarded (Washington, DC: The President's Committee on Mental Retardation, 1969), pp. 255–87; W. Wolfensberger (ed.), *The Principle of Normalisation in Human Services* (Toronto; National Institute of Mental Retardation, 1972).
20. W. Wolfensberger, 'Social Role Valorisation: A Proposed New Term for the Principle of Normalisation', *Mental Retardation*, vol. 21, no. 6 (1983), pp. 234–9.
21. S. Ramon, (ed.), *Beyond Community Care: Normalisation and Integration Work* (London: Macmillan, 1991); H. Brown, and H. Smith (eds), *Normalisation: A Reader for the 1990s* (London: Routledge, 1992).
22. J. McGhee, *Gentle Teaching: A Non-aversive Approach to Helping Persons with Mental Retardation* (Nebraska: Human Sciences Press, 1987).
23. N. Rose and D. Adlam, 'The Subject of Psychiatry: Power, Participation and Resistance', paper presented at the conference 'Psychiatrists' Assumptions: European Philosophy and Pyschiatry', Sheffield, 18–20 September 1992.
24. M. Lawson, 'A Recipient's View', in S. Ramon (ed.), *Beyond Community Care: Normalisation and Integration Work* (London: Macmillan, 1991), pp. 62–84.
25. I. Goffman, *Stigma* (Harmondsworth: Penguin, 1963); T. Scheff, (ed.), *Labelling Madness* (Englewood Cliffs, NJ: Prentice-Hall, 1975); R. Laing, *Self and Others* (London: Tavistock, 1969); D. Cooper, *Psychiatry and Anti-Psychiatry* (London: Tavistock, 1967); K. Dorener, *Madman and the Bourgeoisie* (Oxford: Blackwell, 1979); R. Castel, *The Psychiatric Order* (Cambridge: Polity, 1988); P. Miller and N. Rose (eds), *The Power of Psychiatry* (Cambridge: Polity, 1986); L. Eichenbaum and S. Orbach *Understanding Women* (Harmondsworth: Penguin, 1985); J. Busfield, 'Mental illness as a social product or social construct: a contradiction in Feminists' arguments?', *Sociology of Health and Illness*, vol. 10 (1988), pp. 521–42; S. Fernando, *Mental Health, Race and Culture* (London: Macmillan, 1991).
26. V. Sinason, *Mental Handicap and the Human Condition: New approaches from the Tavistock* (London: Free Association Books, 1992); M. S. Palazoli, L. Boscolo, G. Cecchin and G. Prata, 'Hypothesising, circularity and neutrality: three guidelines for the conductor of the session', *Family Process*, vol. 19 (1980), pp. 45–57; A. T. Beck, *Depression: Clinical, Experimental and Theoretical Aspects* (New York: Harper & Row, 1967).
27. R. Bentall (ed.), *Reconstructing Schizophrenia* (London: Routledge, 1990).
28. L. Ciompi, 'Is there really a schizophrenia: the long term course of psychotic phenomena', *British Journal of Psychiatry*, vol. 145 (1982), pp. 636–640.
29. L. Ciompi, 'Affect Logic: an integrative model of the psyche and its relations to schizophrenia', *British Journal of Psychiatry*, vol. 164, supplement 2 (1994), pp. 51–5.

30. J. Leff and C. Vaughn, *Expressed Emotions in Families* (New York: Guilford, 1985).
31. R. Berkowitz, R. Eberlein-Vries, L. Kupiers and J. Leff, 'Educating Relatives about Schizophrenia', *Schizophrenia Bulletin*, vol. 10 (1984), pp. 418–29.
32. A. T. Beck, A. Rush, B. Shaw and G. Emery, *Cognitive Therapy of Depression* (New York: Guilford, 1979).
33. C. Koettgen and I. Sonninchsen, 'Families high expressed emotions and relapses in young shcizophrenic patients: results of the Hamburg–Camberwell family intervention study', *International Journal of Family Psychiatry*, vol. 5 (1984), pp. 71–82; G. Parker, P. Johnston and L. Hayward, 'Parental expressed emotions as a predictor of schizophrenic relapse', *Archives of General Psychiatry*, vol. 45 (1988), pp. 806–813; L. Barrelet and F. Ferrero, 'Expressed emotions and first admission schizophrenia: a nine months follow-up in a French cultural environment, *British Journal of Psychiatry*, vol. 156 (1990), pp. 357–62.
34. S. Hirsch and J. Leff, *Abnormalities in Parents of Schizophrenics: A review of the literature and an investigation of communication defects and deviances* (Oxford: Oxford University Press, 1975).
35. L. Ciompi, 'Affect Logic', op. cit.
36. G. H. Brown and T. Harris, *The Social Origins of Depression* (London: Macmillan, 1978).
37. E. Ciponi (ed.), *The Treatment of Severe Behavioural Disorders: Behavioural Analysis Approach* (Washington, DC: America Association on Mental Retardation.
38. E. Emerson, S. Barratt, and J. Mansell, *Developing Services for People with Severe Learning Difficulties and Challenging Behaviours* (Canterbury: University of Kent, Institute of Applied Psychology to Social care, 1987).
39. A. H. Reid, 'Prevalence of mental illness among mentally handicapped people', *Journal of the Royal Society of Medicine*, vol. 76 (1984), pp. 587–92.
40. J. Busfield, *Managing Madness* (London: Hutchinson, 1986); S. Ramon, *Psychiatry in Britain: Meaning and Policy* (London: Croom Helm, 1985); S. Ramon, 'The Category of Psychopathy: Its Professional and Social Context in Britain', in P. Miller and N. Rose (eds), *The Power of Psychiatry* (Cambridge: Polity, 1986).
41. M. Romme and S. Escher (eds), *Accepting Voices* (London: Macmillan, 1993).
42. L. J. West, 'Hallucination', in J. W. Howells (ed.), *Modern Perspectives in World Psychiatry* (Edinburgh: Oliver & Boyd, 1968), pp. 265–88; P. Brown, 'Understanding the Inner Voices', *New Scientist*, 9 July 1994, pp. 26–31.
43. Romme and Escher, *Accepting Voices*, op. cit., pp. 6–64.
44. J. Masson, *The Assault on the Truth: Freud's Suppression of the Seduction Theory* (Harmondsworth: Penguin, 1985).
45. See ref. 26; S. Barwick, 'A man in the next bed is not therapeutic', *The Independent*, 5 March 1993; D. Nilbert, S. Cooper and M. Cross-

maker, Assaults against residents of a psychiatric institution: residents history of abuse', *Journal of Interpersonal Violence*, vol. 4, no. 3 (1989), pp. 342–9; V. Sinason, (ed.), *Treating Survivors of Satanic Abuse* (London: Routledge, 1994).

46. A. Cocklin and G. Gorrel-Barnes, 'The shattered picture of the family: encountering new dimensions of human relations of the family and of therapy', in V. Sinason (ed.), *Treating Survivors of Satanic Abuse* (London: Routledge, 1994), pp. 120–30.

47. E. Visard, *Self-esteem and Personal Safety* (London: Tavistock, 1986); D. Finkelhor and A. Browne, 'The traumatic impact of child sexual abuse: a conceptualisation', *American Journal of Orthopsychiatry*, vol. 55 (1985), pp. 530–41.

48. D. Baudin (ed.), *Guide to Mental Health Care in the Netherlands* (Utrecht: The Netherland Institute of Mental Health, 1988).

49. V. Lindow, *Self-Help Alternatives to Mental Health Services* (London: Mind Publications, 1994), pp. 1–10.

50. L. R. Pembroke, (ed.), *Eating Distress: perspectives from personal experience* (London: Survivors Speak Out, 1992).

51. A. Hatfield, *Family Education in Mental Illness* (New York: Guilford, 1990).

52. S. Platt, 'Measuring the burden of psychiatric illness on the family: an evaluation of some rating scales', *Psychological Medicine*, vol. 15 (1986), pp. 383–93; B. McCarthy, 'The Role of Relatives', in A. Lavender and F. Holloway (eds), *Community Care in Practice* (Chichester: Wiley, 1988), pp. 207–27.

53. D. Jones, 'Relative Experience: relatives' experiences of madness', unpublished PhD dissertation, London School of Economics, 1995.

54. N. Garmezy, 'Vulnerability Research and the Issue of Primary Prevention', *American Journal of Orthopsychiatry*, vol. 41, 1971, pp. 101–16.

55. A. Antonovsky, 'Intergenerational Networks and Transmitting the Sense of Coherence', in N. Datan, A. Greene and H. Reese (eds), *Life-span Developmental Psychology: Intergenerational Relations* (Hillsdale, NJ, and London: Lawrence Erlbaum, 1986), pp. 211–23.

56. R. Perske, 'The Dignity of Risk', in W. Wolfensberger (ed.), *The Principle of Normalisation in Human Services* (Toronto, Institute of Mental Retardation, 1979).

57. A. Mullender, A. Everitt, P. Hardiker and J. Littlewood, 'Value Issues in Research', *Social Action*, vol. 1, no. 4 (1993–4), pp. 11–18; C. Argyris and D. A. Schon, *Organisational Learning: a theory of action perspective* (Reading, Mass: Addison-Wesley, 1978); J. O'Brien, 'Embracing Ignorance, Error and Fallibility: competencies for leadership of effective services', in S. Taylor (ed.), *Community Integration* (New York: Teachers College Press of Columbia University, 1987).

58. J. Zeelen, D. van der Meer and W. van de Graaf, 'Action Research in a Psychiatric Hospital', paper presented at the 12th International Science Research Conference, University of Groningen, The Netherlands, 10–14 August 1993.

59. J. Segal, 'The Professional Perspective', in S. Ramon (ed.), *Beyond Community Care: Normalisation and Integration Work* (London: Mac-

millan, 1991), pp. 85–113; D. Brandon, 'Implications of Normalisation Work for Professional Skills', ibid., pp. 35–55.

3 Ethnicity and Gender as Issues for Stakeholders in Mental Distress Services

1. S. Wallman (ed.), *Ethnicity at Work* (London: Macmillan, 1979); V. Saifullah Khan 'The Role of the Culture of Dominance in Structuring the Experience of Ethnic Minorities', in C. Husband, *'Race' in Britain: Continuity and Change* (London: Hutchinson, 1982), pp. 197–215.
2. See L. J. Jordanova, 'Natural Facts: a historical perspective on science and sexuality', in C. MacCormack and M. Strathern (eds), *Nature, Culture and Gender* (Cambridge: Cambridge University Press, 1980); F. Anthias and N. Yuval-Davis, 'Contextualising Feminism – Gender, Ethnic and Class Division', *Feminist Review*, vol. 15 (1983).
3. C. Husband, *'Race' in Britain: Continuity and Change* (London: Hutchinson, 1982); R. Perske, 'The Risk of Dignity', in W. Wolfensberger (ed.) *The Principle of Normalisation in Human Services* (Toronto: Institute of Mental Retardation, 1972), pp. 194–206; S. Kakar, *Shamans Mystics and Doctors: A Psychological Inquiry into India and its Healing Tradition* (London: Allen & Unwin, 1984); S. Fernando, *Mental Health, Race & Culture* (London: Macmillan, 1991); B. Badminter, *The Myth of Motherhood* (London: Souvenir Press, 1980); C. Gilligan, *In a Different Voice: Psychological Theory and Women's Development* (London: Harvard Press, 1982); D. Broverman, F. Clarkson and P. Rosenkratz, 'Sex role stereotypes and clinical judgements of mental health', *Journal of Consulting and Clinical Psychology*, vol. 34, nos 1–7 (1970); E. Showalter, *The Female Malady* (London: Virago, 1987).
4. S. Fernando, *Mental Health, Race & Culture*, op. cit.; D. Pilgrim and A. Rogers, 'Race and Ethnicity', in *A Sociology of Mental Health and Illness* (Buckingham: Open University Press, 1993), pp. 45–62.
5. C. S. Thomas, K. Stone, M. Osborn, P. F. Thomas and M. Fisher, 'Psychiatric Morbidity and Compulsory Admission among UK-born Europeans, Afro-Caribbeans and Asians in Central Manchester', *British Journal of Psychiatry*, vol. 163 (1993), pp. 91–9; R. Cochrene and S. Bal, 'Migration and Schizophrenia: an examination of five hypotheses', *Social Psychiatry*, vol. 22 (1987), pp. 181–91.
6. D. Walsh, 'Psychiatric Care in Ireland', in S. Mangen (ed.) *Mental Health Care in the European Community* (London: Croom Helm, 1985), pp. 148–69.
7. A. Rogers, 'Police and psychiatrists', *Social Policy & Administration*, vol. 27, no. 1 (1993), pp. 33–44.
8. G. Harrison, D. Ownes and A. Holton, 'A prospective study of severe mental disorder in Afro-Caribbean patients', *Psychological Medicine*, vol. 18 (1988), pp. 643–57.

9. C. Thomas et al., 'Psychiatric Morbidity', op. cit.
10. R. Littlewood and M. Lipsedge, *Aliens and Alienists* (Harmondsworth: Penguin, 1982); A Rogers, 'Police and psychiatrists', op. cit.
11. R. Littlewood, 'Ethnic minorities and mental health in Britain: an overview, with some hypotheses for the Greek communities', in N. Bouras and R. Littlewood (eds), *Stress and Coping in the Greek Communities in Britain* (London: Research, Evaluation and Development Unit, Division of Psychiatry, Guy's Hospital, 1988).
12. J. Van Atecum, Psychosomatic disorders in Greeks in the Netherlands', in G. Petrochilos (ed.), *Hellenic Diaspora in Western Europe* (Athens: Vasilopoulos Publishers, 1985); M. V. Piperoglou, 'The Stress of Change: The Greek Migrant Experience', *Australian Family Psychiatry*, vol. 17 (1988), pp. 453–7.
13. C. Bagley, 'The social aetiology of schizophrenia in immigrant groups', *International Journal of Social Psychiatry*, vol. 17 (1971); pp. 292–304, M. Fichter, S. Weyerer and L. Sourdi, 'The epidemiology of anorexia nervosa: a comparison of Greek adolescents living in Germany and Greek adolescents living in Greece', in P. L. Darby (ed.), *Anorexia Nervosa: Recent Developments in Research* (New York: Liss, 1983).
14. E. Francis, 'Black people, dangerousness and psychiatric compulsion', in A. Brackx and C. Grimshaw (eds), *Mental Health Care in Crisis* (London: Pluto 1989); S. Shashidran, 'Ideology and politics in transcultural psychiatry', in J. L. Cox (ed.), *Transcultural Psychiatry* (London: Croom Helm, 1986).
15. F. Fanon, *Black Skin, White Masks* (London: MacGibbon & Kee, 1967).
16. S. Holland, 'Psychotherapy, oppression and social action: gender, race, and class in black women's depression', in R. Perlberg and A. Miller (eds), *Gender and Power in Families* (London: Routledge, 1992), pp. 256–69; E. Francis, 'Black people', op. cit.; S. Shashidran, 'Ideology and Politics', op. cit.
17. S. Holland, 'Psychotherapy', op. cit.; M. M. R. Khan, *When Spring Comes: Awakenings in Psychoanalysis* (London: Chatto & Windus, 1988); J. Kareem and R. Littlewood, *Intercultural Therapy: Themes, Interpretations and Practice* (Oxford: Blackwell, 1993).
18. J. Lewis, (ed.), *Women and Social Policies in Europe* (Aldershot: Edward Elgar, 1993), p. 11.
19. A. Oakley, 'Normal Motherhood: an exercise in self control?', in B. Hutter and G. Williams (eds), *Controlling Women: The Normal and the Deviant* (London: Croom Helm, 1981); S. Walby, *Patriarchy at Work: Patriarchal and Capitalist Relations in Employment* (London: Polity, 1989); H. Graham, 'Coping: or how mothers are seen and not heard', in S. Friedman and E. Sarah (eds), *On the Problem of Men* (London: The Women's Press, 1982).
20. L. Diamont, *Male and Female Homosexuality: Psychological Approaches* (New York: Hemisphere, 1987).
21. M. Barnes and N. Maple, *Women and Mental Health: Challenging the Stereotypes* (Birmingham: Venture Press, 1992); M. Kastrup, 'Sex

differences in the utilization of mental health services: a nationwide register study', *International Journal of Social Psychiatry*, vol. 33, no. 3 (1987), pp. 171–84.
22. M. Barnes and N. Maple, 'Later Life – Old Age', in M. Barnes and N. Maple, *Women and Mental Health*, pp. 97–120; S. Platt, 'Unemployment and suicidal behaviour: a review of the literature', *Social Science and Medicine*, vol. 19 (1984), pp. 93–115; P. Crept and F. Lofrenzano, 'Unemployment and suicide in Italy', in H. J. Moller (ed.), *Current Issues of Suicidology* (Berlin: Springer, 1988).
23. V. Svab-Cotic, 'Continued Care Clients in Slovenia', *International Journal of Social Psychiatry*, vol. 40, no. 4 (1994).
24. J. Busfield, 'Gender and Mental Illness', *International Journal of Mental Health*, vol. 11, nos 1–2 (1982), pp. 46–66; M. G. Cogliati, S. Petri and M. T. Pini, 'Gender in the Italian Services', in S. Ramon (ed.), *Psychiatry in Transition* (London: Pluto, 1990), pp. 99–108; L. Eichenbaum and S. Orbach, *Outside In Inside Out* (Harmondsworth: Penguin, 1982).
25. V. Nice, *Mothers & Daughters: The Distortion of a Relationship* (London: Macmillan, 1992). S. Macintyre, *Single and Pregnant* (London: Croom Helm, 1977).
26. M. Sheppard, 'General practice, social work and mental health sections: the social control of women', *British Journal of Social Work*, vol. 21 (1991), pp. 663–83; A. Davis, S. P. Llewellyn and G. Parry, 'Women and mental health: a guide for the approved social worker', in E. Broom and A. Davis (eds), *Women, the Family and Social Work* (London: Tavistock, 1985).
27. L. Johnstone, *Users and Abusers of Psychiatry* (London: Routledge, 1989), pp. 100–26.
28. N. Rose, *The Psychological Complex* (London: Blackwell, 1985); S. Ramon, *Psychiatry in Britain: Meaning and Policy* (London: Croom Helm, 1985).
29. S. Fenton and A. Sadiq, *Asian Women and Depression* (London: Commission for Racial Equality, 1991).
30. M. Lawrence, *The Anorexic Experience* (London: The Women's Press, 1984); L. Pembroke (ed.), *Eating Distress: Perspectives from Personal Experience* (London: Survivors Speak Out, 1992).
31. R. Jack, *Women and Attempted Suicide* (London: Lawrence Erlbaum, 1992).
32. L. Pembroke, *Eating Distress*, op. cit.; V. Lindow, 'Experts, Lies and Stereotypes', *The Health Service Journal*, 29 August 1991, pp. 18–19; V. Lindow, *Self Help Alternatives and Mental Health Services* (London: Mind Publications, 1994).
33. T. Gray and L. Swindell, *Young women's sexual abuse group evaluation report* (London: Greenwich Social Services and Thamesmead Family Service Unit, 1987).
34. R. E. Perkins and L. A. Rowland, 'Sex-differences in service usage in long term psychiatric care – are women adequately served', *British Journal of Psychiatry*, vol. 158, S10 (1991), pp. 75–9.
35. G. Dalley, *Ideologies of Caring* (London: Macmillan, 1988); J. Lewis

and B. Meredith, *Daughters who Care: Daughters Caring for Mothers at Home* (London: Routledge, 1988); P. Chamberlayne, 'Care Cultures: The Case of the Two Germanies', paper presented at the conference on 'international perspectives of health social work in the 1990', 4 July 1994, London School of Economics.
36. M. O'Brien, 'The Place of Men in Gender-Sensitive Therapy', in R. Perlberg and A. Miller (eds), *Gender and Power in Families* (London: Routledge, 1992), pp. 195–208.
37. M. Briscoe, 'Sex differences in psychological well-being', *Psychological Medicine Monograph Supplement 1* (Cambridge: Cambridge University Press, 1982); K. Solomon, 'Individual psychotherapy and changing masculine roles: dimensions of gender-role psychotherapy', in K. Solomon and N. Levy (eds), *Men in Transition: Theory and Therapy* (New York: Plenum, 1982).
38. M. Brearly, 'Counsellors and clients: men or women', *Marriage Guidance*, vol. 22, no 2 (1986), pp. 3–9; L. A. Kirchner, S. T. Hauser and A. Genack, 'Research on gender and psychotherapy', in M. T. Notman and C. C. Nadlsen (eds), *The Woman Patient* (New York: 1982).
39. P. Crepet, *Le Dimensioni del Vuoto: i giovani e il suicidio* (Rome: Fletrinelli, 1994); K. Hawton, *Suicide and Attempted Suicide among Children and Adolescents* (Beverly Hills: Sage, 1986).
40. C. Pritchard, 'Is There a Link between Suicide in Young Men and Unemployment? A Comparison of the UK with other European Community Countries', *British Journal of Psychiatry*, vol. 160 (1992), pp. 750–756.
41. S. Platt, 'Unemployment and suicidal behaviour: a review of the literature', *Social Science and Medicine*, vol. 19 (1984), pp. 93–115.
42. M. Lawrence, *The Anorexic Experience*, op. cit.
43. J. Williams, G. Watson, H. Smith, J. Cooperman and D. Wood, *Purchasing Effective Mental Health Services for Women: A Framework for Action* (Canterbury: University of Kent, 1993).
44. A. Mullender and D. Ward, *Self-directed Groupwork* (London: Whiting & Birch, 1991).
45. B. Knight, *Family Groups in the Community* (London: Voluntary Service Council, 1979); S. Holland, 'The development of an action and counselling service in a deprived urban area', in M. Meacher (ed.), *New Methods of Mental Health Care* (Oxford: Pergamon, 1979); S. Holland, 'Towards Prevention', in S. Ramon (ed.), *Psychiatry in Transition* (London: Pluto, 1990), pp. 125–37.
46. R. Perlberg and A. Miller (eds), *Gender and Power in Families* (London: Routledge, 1992).
47. R. Hare-Mustin, 'A feminist approach to family therapy', in E. Howell and M. Bayes (eds), *Women and Mental Health* (New York: Basic Books, 1981).
48. B. Mason, 'Neutrality: the worker and family therapy', in M. Marshall, M. Preston-Shoot and E. Wincott (eds), *Skills for Social Workers in the 1980s* (Birmingham: British Association of Social Workers, 1986).

49. G. H. Brown and T. Harris, *The Social Origins of Depression* (London: Macmillan, 1978).
50. R. Corney and R. Jenkins, *Counselling in Primary Care* (London: Routledge, 1993).

4 Long-Term Users of Mental Health Services

1. G. Thornicroft, D. Jones and O. Margolious, 'New Long Stay Psychiatric Patients and Social Deprivation', *British Journal of Psychiatry*, vol. 161 (1992), pp. 621–4.
2. R. Warner, *Recovery from Schizophrenia* (London: Routledge, 1985).
3. J. K. Wing and R. Furlong, 'A Haven to the Severely Disabled within the Context of Comprehensive Psychiatric Community Service', *British Journal of Psychiatry*, vol. 149 (1986), pp. 449–57.
4. M. Jones, *Social Psychiatry* (London: Tavistock, 1952).
5. M. Levander, 'The Context of Chronic Patients', *Acta Psychiatrica Scandinavica*, vol. 77 (1987), p. 26.
6. J. Lacan, 'Le stade du mirror comme formateur de la fonction de Je', in *Ecrits* (Paris: Editions du Seuil, 1966); F. Guattari, *Molecular Revolution: Psychiatry and Politics* (Harmondsworth: Penguin, 1984); G. Deleuze and F. Guattari, *Anti-Aedipus: Capitalism and Schizophrenia* (New York: Viking, 1977); M. Cadoret, L'enfant et l'adolescent, pratique instutionnelle publique: une question d'ethique et de responsibilite, in C. Louzoun (ed.), *Sante Mentale: Realites Europeennes* (Paris: Eres, 1993), pp. 80–2.
7. N. Scheper-Huges and A. Lovell, *In and Out of Psychiatry: Selections from Franco Basaglia's Writings* (New York: Columbia University Press, 1987); F. Rotelli, 'Changing Psychiatric Services in Italy', in S. Ramon (ed.), *Psychiatry in Transition* (London: Pluto, 1990), pp. 182–90; S. Piro, *Le Techniche della Liberazione* (Rome, Feltrineeli, 1971).
8. G. De Plato (ed.), 'Cos'e la Riabilitazione in Psichiatria? Pordenone', *Medicina Sociale 2* (Edizioni Biblioteca dell'Immagine, 1993).
9. B. Saraceno, 'La riaiblitazione fra modelli e pratiche', in G. De Plato, 'Cos'e la Riabilitazione in Psichiodria', op. cit., pp. 35–48.
10. C. Brooker (ed.), *Community Psychiatric Nursing: A Research Perspective* (London: Chapman and Hall, 1990); M. Savio, 'Psychiatric Nursing in Italy: An extinguished profession or an emerging professionalism?', *International Journal of Social Psychiatry*, vol. 37, no. 4 (1991), pp. 293–9.
11. P. Tranchina, E. Salvi, M. P. Teodori and S. Rogialli (eds), *Portelano della Psicologia: Esperienze, prospettive, convergenze di una professione giovane* (Pistoia: Cooperative Centro di Documentazione, 1993).
12. V. Sinason, *The Sense in Stupidity: Psychotherapy and Mental Handicap* (London: Free Associations, 1992).
13. H. Brown and H. Smith (eds), *Normalisation: A Reader for the 1990s* (London: Routledge, 1992).

14. S. Shardlow (ed.), *Values for Change in Social Work* (London: Heinmann, 1989); W. Lorenz, *Social Work in a Changing Europe* (London: Routledge, 1993).
15. S. Ramon, *Mental Health Social Workers' Responses to the 1990 NHS and Community Care Act* (Birmingham: BASW, September 1993); R. Rachman, 'Health Social Workers' reactions to the NHS and Community Care Act', paper presented to the conference 'International Trends in Health Social Work', London School of Economics, 4–8 July 1994.
16. B. McCarthy, L. Kuipers, J. Hurry, R. Harper and A. Lesage, 'Counselling the Relatives of the Long-term Adult mentally Ill', *British Journal of Psychiatry*, vol. 154 (1989), pp. 768–75; A. Hatfield, *Family Education in Mental Illness* (New York: Guildford, 1990); S. Deacon, 'It is Chris's illness but we all have the scars', *The Independent*, 2 January 1992.
17. D. Jones, 'Relative Experience of Schizophrenia', PhD thesis, London School of Economics, 1995.
18. European User Network, First Conference of Users and Ex-users in Mental Health, Zandvoort, the Netherlands, October 1991; published by the European Desk, Amsterdam.
19. A. Lavender and F. Holloway (eds), *Community Care in Practice*, Section A. Introduction (Chichester: Wiley, 1988), pp. 3–50.
20. J. Yfantopolous, 'Economic and Legal Aspects of Mental Health Policies in Greece', *International Journal of Social Psychiatry*, vol. 40, no. 4 (1994).
21. V. Svab, 'Continuing Care Clients in Slovenia', *International Journal of Social Psychiatry*, vol. 40, no. 4 (1994).
22. T. Grove, 'Who needs long term psychiatric care?', *British Medical Journal*, vol. 300 (1990), pp. 999–1001.
23. L. Ciompi, 'Aging and Schizophrenic Psychosis', *Acta Psychiatrica Scandinavica*, supplement 319, vol. 71 (1985), pp. 93–105.
24. C. McCourt Perring, 'The experience and perspectives of patients and care staff on the transition from hospital to community-based care', in S. Ramon (ed.), *Psychiatric Hospitals Closure: Myths and Realities* (London: Chapman & Hall, 1992), pp. 122–68.
25. C. Strutti and S. Rauber, 'Leros and the Greek Mental Health system', *International Journal of Social Psychiatry*, vol. 40, no. 4 (1994).
26. R. G. McCreadie and E. McCannell, 'The Scottish Survey of New Chronic In-patients: Five-year Follow-up, *British Journal of Psychiatry*, vol. 155 (1989), pp. 348–51.
27. J. Reed, *Review of Health and Social Services for Mentally Disordered Offenders and others Requiring Similar Services* (London: Department of Health, HMSO, 1991); R. Mezzina, 'Le travail des services psychiatriques a la prison de Trieste: principles, realites', in C. Louzoun (ed.) *Sante Mentale: Realites Europeannes* (Paris: Eres, 1993), pp. 289–300.
28. C. Revon, 'La place, le role, la responsiblite de l'avocat ayant en charge de defense d'un malade mentale une juridiction penale', in C. Louzoun (ed.), *Sante Mentale*, op. cit., pp. 280–3.

29. *Social Work in Europe*, vol. 1, no. 1 (Russell House Publishing), p. 35.
30. S. Bell, G. Robertson, K. James and A. Grounds, 'Remands and Psychiatric Assessments in Holloway Prison: i: The Psychotic Population', *British Journal of Psychiatry*, vol. 163 (1993), pp. 634–40.
31. P. Joseph and M. Potter, 'Diversion from Custody: I: Psychiatric Assessment at the Magistrates' Court', *British Journal of Psychiatry*, vol. 162 (1993), pp. 325–30; P. Joseph and M. Potter, 'Diversion from Custody: II: Effect on Hospital and Prison Resources', *British Journal of Psychiatry*, vol. 162 (1993), pp. 330–4.
32. Mental Health Act Commission: The Ashworth Special Hospital Inquiry (London: HMSO, 1992).
33. 'A Research Agenda for Women and Special Hospitals', workshop held at Ashworth Special Hospital, 21 January, 1993.
34. WISH Monologue, based on the collective experience of women in Ashworth, prepared for the meeting on 'Women in Special Hospitals: A research agenda', 21 January 1993, Ashworth.
35. G. Del Guidice, 'The Judicial Psychiatric Hospital: A Difficult Reform?', in S. Ramon (ed.), *Psychiatry in Transition* (London: Pluto, 1990), pp. 157–65; R. Mezzina, 'Le travail des services psychiatriques', op. cit.
36. A. Rogers, D. Pilgrim and R. Lacey, *Experiencing Psychiatry: Users' Views of Services* (London: Macmillan, 1993).
37. C. McCourt Perring, 'The experience and perspectives of patients and care staff', op. cit.; M. Knapp, J. Beecham and P. Cambridge, *Community Care: The Challenge* (Canterbury: University of Kent, Personal Social Services Research Unit, 1992); D. Dayson, 'Long-stay patients discharged to the community: Followed-up at 1, 2 and 5 years', TAPS (team for the assessment of psychiatric services), 9th Annual Conference, 21 July 1994.
38. T. Wykes and J. K. Wing, ' "New" long-stay patients: the nature and size of the problem', in R. Young (ed.), *Residential Needs of Severely Disabled Psychiatric Patients – The Case for Hospital Hostels* (London: HMSO, 1991).
39. P. Mortensen and K. Juel, 'Mortality and Causes of Death in First Admitted Schizophrenic Patients', *British Journal of Psychiatry*, vol. 163 (1993), pp. 183–9.
40. M. Birchwood, R. Cochrane, F. Macmillan, D. Copestake, J. Kucharska and M. Cariss, 'The Influence of Ethnicity and Family Structure on Relapse in First-episode Schizophrenia: A Comparison of Asian, Afro-Caribbean and White Patients', *British Journal of Psychiatry*, vol. 161 (1992), pp. 783–90.
41. HMSO Report of the Inquiry into the Care and Treatment of Christopher Clunis (the Ritchie Report) (London: HMSO, 1994); L. Blom-Cooper, H. Hally and E. Murphy, *The Falling shadow: One Patient's Mental Health Care 1978–1993* (London: Duckworth, 1995).
42. V. Hiday and T. Scheid-Cook, 'A Follow-up of Chronic Patients Committed to Outpatient Treatment', *Hospital and Community Psychiatry*, vol. 40, no. 1 (1989), pp. 52–8; Department of Health, *Legal Powers on the Care of Mentally Ill People in the Community: Report of the*

Internal Review (London: HMSO, 1993); Department of Health, *Guidance on the Discharge of Mentally Disordered People and their Continuing Care in the Community* (London: DoH, HSG (94) 27, 1994).
43. M. Lawrence, *The Anorexic Experience* (London: The Women's Press, 1984); Secretary of State for Health, *The Health of the Nation* (London: HMSO, 1991); G. Thonicroft and G. Strathdee, 'Mental Health', *British Medical Journal*, vol. 303, (17 August 1991), pp. 41–42; L. R. Pembroke, *Self-Harm: Perspectives from Personal Experience* (London: Survivors Speak Out, 1994).
44. Ibid.
45. R. D. Scott, 'A family oriented psychiatric service to the London Borough of Barnet', *Health Trends*, vol. 12 (1980); pp. 65–8; S. Onyett, P. Tryer and J. Conolly, 'The Early Intervention Service: the first 18 months of an inner London demonstration project', *Psychiatric Bulletin*, vol. 14 (1990), pp. 276–9.
46. C. Louzoun (ed.), *Sante Mentale: Realites Europennes* (Paris: Eres, 1993); L. Mosher and L. Burti (eds), *Community Mental Health: Principles and Practice* (New York: Norton, 1989); S. Morgan, *Community Mental Health: Practical approaches to long-term problems* (London: Chapman & Hall, 1993).
47. M. D. Farkas, 'Care Innovation Projects: Issues in Rehabilitation', in J. Wolf and J. van Weeghel (eds), *Changing Community Psychiatry: Care Innovation for Persons with Long-Term Mental Illness in the Netherlands*, (Utrecht: The Netherlands Institute of Mental Health, 1993), pp. 63–88.
48. M. Piccinelli and G. Wilkinson, 'Outcome of Depression in Psychiatric Settings: Review Article', *British Journal of Psychiatry*, vol. 164 (1994), pp. 297–304.
49. J. A. Lieberman, 'Understanding the mechanism of action of atypical antipsychotic drugs: A review of compounds in the use and development, in D. Addington and J. Addington (eds), 'The Psychopharmacology of Schizophrenia', *The British Journal of Psychiatry*, vol. 163, Supplement 22 (December 1993), pp. 7–18.
50. D. Addington and J. Addington, 'The Psychopharmacology of Schizophrenia', op. cit., p. 6.
51. S. G. Siris, 'Adjunctive medication in the maintenance treatment of schizophrenia and its conceptual implications', in D. Addington and J. Addington, 'The Psychopharmacology of Schizophrenia', op. cit., pp. 66–78.
52. P. Breggin, *Toxic Psychiatry* (New York: Fontana, 1985).
53. F. Holloway, 'Prescribing for the long-term mentally ill: a study of treatment practice', *British Journal of Psychiatry*, vol. 149 (1988); pp. 75–81; M. Muijen and T. Silverstone, 'A comparative hospital survey of psychotropic drugs prescribing', *British Journal of Psychiatry*, vol. 150 (1987), pp. 501–4.
54. T. Cantopher, S. Olivieri, N. Cleave and J. G. Edwards, 'Chronic Benzodiazepine Dependence: A comparative study of abrupt withdrawal after Popranolol cover vs. gradual withdrawal', *British*

Journal of Psychiatry, vol. 156 (1990); pp. 406–11; P. Jenkinson, 'Gradual withdrawal of major tranquillisers', paper presented to the diploma course: Innovation in Mental Health Work, February 1994.
55. J. Masson, *Against Therapy* (New York: Fontana, 1988).
56. V. Sinason, The Sense in Stupidity, op. cit.; R. Perlberg, and A. Miller (eds), *Gender and Power in Families* (London: Routledge, 1992); P. Janssen, 'The Evolution of Inpatient Psychoanalytic Therapy in Germany', *Therapeutic Communities*, vol. 14, no. 4 (1993), pp. 265–74; A. Ryle, *Cognitive Analytic Therapy* (Chichester: Wiley, 1991).
57. V. Sinason, *The Sense in Stupidity*, op. cit.; V. Sinason (ed.), *Treating Survivors of Satanist Abuse* (London: Routledge, 1994); A. Higgitt and P. Fonagy, 'Psychotherapy in Borderline and Narcissistic Personality Disorder', *British Journal of Psychiatry*, Review Article, vol. 161 (1992), pp. 23–43.
58. R. Warner, 'Creative Programming', in S. Ramon (ed.), *Beyond Community Care: Normalisation and Integration Work* (London: Macmillan, 1991), pp. 114–36; L. Stein and M. A. Test, (eds), *The Training in Community Living Model: A Decade of Experience, New Directions for Mental Health Service 26* (San Francisco: Joseey-Bass).
59. M. Muijen, I. Marks and J. Connolly, 'The Daily Living Programme: Preliminary comparison of community vs. hospital-based treatment for the seriously mentally ill facing emergency admission', *British Journal of Psychiatry*, vol. 160 (1992); pp. 379–84; M. Muijen, I. Marks and J. Connolly, 'Home based care and standard hospital care for patients with severe mental illness: a randomised control trial', *British Medical Journal*, vol. 304 (1992), pp. 749–54.
60. B. McCarthy, 'The Role of Relatives', in A. Lavender and F. Holloway (eds) *Community Care in Practice* (Chichester: Wiley, 1988), pp. 207–30; I. Falloon, *Managing Stress in Families: Cognitive and Behavioural Strategies for Enhancing Coping Skills* (London: Routledge, 1993).
61. D. Howe, *The Consumer View of Family Therapy* (Aldershot: Gower, 1989).
62. S. Onyett, *Case Management in Mental Health* (London: Chapman Hall, 1992).
63. J. Wolf, and J. van Weeghel (eds), *Changing Community Psychiatry: Care Innovation for Persons with Long-term Mental Illness in the Netherlands* (Utrecht: The Netherlands Institute of Mental Health, 1993).
64. J. K. Wing (ed.), *The Evaluation of Comprehensive Community Psychiatric Services* (Oxford: Oxford University Press, 1972).
65. L. Doyal and I. Gough, *A Theory of Human Needs* (London: Macmillan, 1993); C. A. Rapp and R. Wintersteen, 'The Strengths Model of Case Management: results from twelve demonstrations', *Psychosocial Rehabilitation Journal*, vol. 13, no. 1 (1989), pp. 23–32.
66. J. Wolf and J. van Weeghel, *Changing Community Psychiatry*, op. cit., see also reference 46.
67. D. Brandon and N. Towe, *Free to Choose* (London: Good Impressions, 1989); D. Brandon, 'Skills for Service Brokerage', in S. Ramon

(ed.), *Care Management: Implications for Training* (Sheffield: Association of Teachers in Social Work Education, 1992), pp. 60–5.
68. A. Hatfield, 'The National Alliance for the Mentally Ill: The Meaning of a Movement', *International Journal of Mental Health*, vol. 4 (1987), pp. 79–93.
69. P. Arksey, 'The Support of the National Schizophrenia Fellowship to Relatives', paper presented at the conference 'Opening the Dialogue', London School of Economics, January 1992.
70. See D. Baudin (ed.), *A Guide to Mental Health Care in the Netherlands* (Utrecht: The Netherlands Institute of Mental Health, 1988), pp. 55–6.
71. L. Soglia, 'L'esperienza di Associazione di familiari, degenti e operator', in G. De Plato (ed.), 'Cos'e la Riabilitazione in Psychiatria? Pordenone', *Medicina Sociale* (Edizioni Biblioteca dell'Imagine), vol. 2 (1993), pp. 183–8.
72. J. Chamberlin, *On Our Own* (London: Mind Publications, 1989).
73. D. Baudin, *A Guide to Mental Health Care*, chapter 3: 'Clients and Organisations'; M. O'Hagan, *Stopovers on my way home from Mars: A journey into the psychiatric survivors movement in the USA, Britain and the Netherlands* (London: Survivors Speak Out, 1993).
74. E. Van Horn, 'Changes? What Changes? The view of the European Patients' Movement', *International Journal of Psychiatry*, vol. 38, no. 1 (1992), pp. 30–5.
75. European User Network First European Conference of Users and Ex-users in Mental Health, Zandvoort, The Netherlands, October 1991, published by the European Desk, Amsterdam; European Regional Council, *World Mental Health Federation: The Mental Health Observer/L'observateur en Sante Mentale*, vol. 6 (Brussels, European Regional Council, Autumn 1994).
76. The Prato self-help group can be contacted at AISME (Associazione Italiana Salute Mentale), Sede legale Via Livi, Prato Cap 50047, Italy.
77. J. Wallcraft and S. Bell (eds) *Survivors Speak Out News Sheet* (London: SSO) August, 1994.
78. V. Lindow, *Self-help Alternatives to Mental Health Services* (London: Mind Publications, 1994).
79. V. Lindow, 'Survivor, Activist, or Witch', *Asylum Magazine for Democratic Psychiatry*, (Sheffield), vol. 7, no. 4 (1993), pp. 5–7.
80. E. van Hoorn, 'Changes? What changes?', op. cit.

5 Innovations in Housing and Employment

1. D. Brandon, 'Homelessness: the way ahead', *Community Care*, 1974, pp. 16–19; W. A. Hamid, T. Wykes and S. Stansfield. 'The Homeless Mentally Ill: Myths and Realities', *International Journal of Social Psychiatry*, vol. 39, no. 4 (1993), pp. 237–54.

2. J. Scott, 'Homelessness and Mental Illness: Review Article', *British Journal of Psychiatry*, vol. 162 (1993), pp. 314–24.
3. K. Bhoi, 'Brixton Court Diversion Scheme', paper presented at the conference 'Our Special Hospitals', London School of Economics, 12 December 1993.
4. M. O'Neill, *Users of Resettlement Units: a report of a survey carried out in fifteen Resettlement Units and a census carried out in all twenty-two* (London: Resettlement Agency, 1989).
5. J. Scott, 'Homelessness and Mental Illness', op. cit.
6. T. Wykes, 'A hostel-ward for "new" long stay patients', in J. K. Wing (ed.), 'Long-Term Community Care', *Psychological Medicine*, Supplement 2 (1982), pp. 41–55.
7. J. Maguire, *A Hospital–Hostel Based on the Principle of Normalisation* (London: Innovation Project Report, Diploma Innovation in Mental Health Work, London School of Economics, 1994).
8. D. Mauri (ed.), *La Liberta E Terapeutica?* (Rome: Feltrinelli, 1986); R. Mezzina, P. Mazzuia, D. Vidoni and M. Impagnatiello, 'Networking consumers' participation in a communal mental health service: mutual support groups, "citizenship", coping strategies', *International Journal of Social Psychiatry*, vol. 38, no. 1 (1992), pp. 68–73; P. Tranchina and P. Serra, 'Community Work and Participation in the New Italian Psychiatric Legislation', in H. Stierlin (ed.), *Psychological Intervention and Schizophrenia: An International View* (New York: Springer Verlag, 1982), pp. 109–20.
9. E. Roosnes, *The Mad in the Town: Gheel and its secular therapy* (London: Sage, 1979).
10. D. Jodelet, *Social Representations of Madness* (Hemel Hampstead; Wheatsheaf, 1991).
11. Ibid., p. 35.
12. Ibid., p. 39.
13. Ibid., p. 268.
14. Ibid., p. 274.
15. L. Tagliabue, 'Riflessioni sulla practica delle structure intermedie a Reggio Emilia', in G. De Plato (ed.), *Cose' la riabilitazione in Psychiatria?* (Pordenone: Medicina Sociale, 1993), pp. 141–50.
16. R. Mezzina, P. Mazzuia, D. Vidoni and M. Imapgnatiello, 'Networking consumers' participation in a community mental health service: mutual support groups, "citizenship", coping strategies', *International Journal of Social Psychiatry*, vol. 38, no. 1 (1992), pp. 68–73.
17. C. McCourt Perring, 'The experience and perspectives of patients and care staff on the transition from hospital to community-based care', in S. Ramon (ed.), *Psychiatric Hospitals Closure: Myths and Realities* (London: Chapman & Hall, 1992), pp. 122–68.
18. A. Petch, *A Home in the Community: An evaluation of supported accommodation for people with mental health problems* (Aldershot: Avebury, 1993); M. Knapp, P. Cambridge, C. Thomason, J. Beecham, C. Allen and R. Darton, *Care in the Community? Challenge and Demonstration* (Aldershot: Avebury, 1992); C. Crosby, M. M. Barry, M. F. Carter

and J. Bogg, *Evaluation of Resettlement from North Wales Hospital: Brief Report on the Care Process in Two Community Care Schemes* (Bangor: Health Services Research Unit, University of North Wales, 1992); TAPS (Team for the Assessment of Psychiatric Services) *Better Out Than In?* (London: North East Thames Regional health Authority, 1990).
19. M. Knapp and J. Beecham, 'Costing psychiatric interventions', in G. Thornicroft, C. Berwin and J. K. Wing, *Measuring Mental Health Needs* (London: Gaskell, 1992).
20. B. Schumacher, *Doing Away with Night Cover*, Innovation Project Report (London: Diploma in Innovation in Mental Health Work, London School of Economics, 1990), and personal communication 1993.
21. C. Gell and N. Prance, 'Service Development in Housing', London study day on 'Achieving Innovation in Mental Health Services', Pavilion, 7 July 1994.
22. E. Karkoff, 'Community Services for the Chronically Mentally Ill in the FRG (Federal German Republic)', in R. Hollingworth and E. Hollingworth (eds), *Services for the Severely Ill* (New York: Aldine de Gruyter, 1994); see also reference 14.
23. Petch, *A Home in the Community*.
24. Ibid., pp. 162, 166.
25. Ibid., p. 163.
26. A. Kay and C. Legg, *Discharged to the Community: a review of housing and support in London for people leaving psychiatric care* (London: City University, 1986); A. Rogers, D. Pilgrim and R. Lacey, *Experiencing Psychiatry: Users' Views of Services* (London: Macmillan, 1993).
27. P. Warr, *Work, Unemployment and Mental Health* (Oxford: Oxford University Press, 1984); L. Fagin, and M. Little, *The Foresaken Families* (Harmondsworth: Penguin, 1982).
28. J. Mattinson, and I. Sinclair, *Mate and Stalemate* (London: Tavistock, 1989).
29. E. Karkoff, 'Community Services', op. cit.
30. S. Pilling, *Rehabilitation and Community Care* (London: Routledge, 1992); E. Murphy, *After the Asylum* (London: Longman, 1993).
31. A. Birch, *What Chance Have We Got? Occupation & Employment after Mental Illness – Patients' Views* (Manchester: Mind in Manchester, 1983).
32. G. Shepherd, 'Psychiatric Rehabilitation for the 1990s', in F. N. Watts and D. H. Bennett (eds), *Theory and Practice of Psychiatric Rehabilitation* (Chichester: Wiley, 1991).
33. A. Kay and C. Legg, *Discharged to the Community*, op. cit.; A. Rogers et al., *Experiencing Psychiatry*, op. cit.
34. M. De Jonge, *Gek(k)en Werk*. Lezing op het arbeidsrehabilitatiecongress, Maastricht, 20 April 1989, as quoted in J. Zeelen and J. van Weeghel, *Vocational Rehabilitation in a Changing Psychiatry* (Groningen: Department of Andragology, 1993).
35. R. Warner, 'Building Programmes', in S. Ramon, (ed.), *Beyond*

Community Care: Normalisation and Integration Work (London: Macmillan, 1991); see also reference 8.
36. J. Beard, R. Propost and T. Malamud, 'The Fountain House Model of Psychiatric Rehabilitation', *Psychosocial Rehabilitation Journal*, vol. 5 (1982), pp. 47–53; J. Nehring, R. Hill and L. Poole, 'Hillside House, the first British Club House', in *Work, Employment and Community: Opportunities for people with long-term mental health problems* (London: Research and Development in Psychiatry, 1993), pp. 13–20.
37. N. Winston, London, Diploma Innovation in Mental Health Work, Innovation Project Report, 1994.
38. J. Zeelen and J. van Weeghel, *Vocational Rehabilitation in a Changing Psychiatry* (Groningen: Department of Andragology, 1993).
39. K. Tudor, 'The Politics of Disability in Italy: La lega per il Diritto al lavoro degli Handicappati', *Critical Social Policy*, 1988, pp. 37–54.
40. G. Room (ed.), *Anti-poverty Action-Research in Europe* (Bristol: School for Advanced Urban Studies, 1993).
41. O. De Leonardis, D. Mauri and F. Rotelli, *L'impresa Sociale* (Milan: Anabasi, 1994).
42. M. Savio and A. Righetti, 'Cooperatives as a social enterprise in Italy: a place for social intergration and rehabilitation', *Acta Psychiatrica Scandinavica*, vol. 88 (1993), pp. 238–42; O. De Leonardis, *et al.*, L'impresa Sociale, op. cit., S. Ramon, 'The Work Cooperatives in Trieste: A Case Study of Immersion in the Community', in R. Schulz and J. Greenley (eds), *Implementing Change for Community Care for Persons with Severe Mental Illness* (New York: Praeger, 1995).
43. M. T. Battaglino and A. Di Maschio (eds), *Volevamo Soltanto Cambiare il Mondo* (Turin: Edizioni Sonda, 1992); A. Di Mascio, 'L'esperienza della Nuova cooperativa nel processo di superamento del Ospedale Psichiatrico', paper presented at the conference 'Commincare di Essere', Villa Gualino, Turin, USL 24, 16 December 1993.
44. A. Righetti, M. Savio and G. Weber, 'Valutazione della funzione riabilitativa e di integrazione sociale dell'impresa sociale 'Coop Service Noncello', *Medicina Sociale Epidemiologia* (Pordenone), vol. 3 (1994), pp. 83–96.

6 Changing Professional Roles and Identities

1. R. Dingwall and P. Lewis (eds), *The Sociology of the Professions* (London: Macmillan, 1983).
2. T. Johnson, *Professions and Power* (London: Macmillan, 1972); A. Witz, 'Patriarchy and Professions: The Gendered Politics of Occupational Closure', *Sociology*, vol. 24, no. 4 (1990), pp. 675–90.
3. P. Nolan, *A History of Mental Health Nursing* (London: Chapman Hall, 1993); M. Savio, 'Pathways to Professionalism: The Development of Community Psychiatric Nursing in Britain and Italy', unpublished PhD thesis (London School of Economics, 1994).

4. E. Freidson, *Professional Powers: A Study of Institutionalisation of Formal Knowledge* (Chicago: University of Chicago Press, 1986).
5. Freedom to Care, *The Whistle*, no. 5 (West Molesey, Surrey: Freedom to Care, September 1994).
6. D. Towell and T. Macausland, *Managing Psychiatric Services in Transition: An overview* (London: King Edward Hospital Fund for London, 1988).
7. L. Carrino and S. Petri, 'Community Action in Giugliano', *Community Development Journal*, vol. 19, no. 2 (1984), pp. 88–95; S. Morgan, *Community Mental Health: Practical approaches to long-term problems* (London: Chapman & Hall, 1993); S. Trevellion, *Caring in the Community: a network approach to community partnership* (London: Longman, 1992).
8. S. Morgan, *Community Mental Health*, op. cit., pp. 53–61; C. A. Rapp and R. Wintersteen, 'The Strengths Model of Case Management: results from twelve demonstrations', *Psychosocial Rehabilitation Journal*, vol. 13, no. 1, pp. 23–32.
9. D. Jones, D. Tomlinson and J. Anderson, 'Asylums and Community Care: plus change', *Journal of the Royal Society of Medicine*, vol. 84, pp. 252–4; A. Jablonsky, 'Politics and Mental Health I' and F. Basaglia-Ongaro, 'Politics and Mental Health II', *International Journal of Social Psychiatry*, vol. 38, no. 1 (1992), pp. 24–30, 36–40.
10. P. Owen, H. Glennerster and M. Matsganis, *Implementing Fundholding in General Practice* (Milton Keynes: The Open University, 1994).
11. M. Knapp, P. Cambridge, J. Beecham, C. Allen and R. Darton, *Care in the Community: Challenge and Demonstration* (Canterbury: Personal Social Services Research Unit, University of Kent, 1992).
12. D. Brandon, *Innovation without Change?* (London: Macmillan, 1991); D. Brandon and N. Towe, *Free to Choose* (London: Good Impressions, 1990).
13. C. McCourt Perring, 'The Experience and perspectives of patients and care staff on the transition from hospital to community-based care, in S. Ramon (ed.), *Psychiatric Hospital Closure: Myths and Realities* (London: Chapman & Hall, 1992), pp. 122–68.
14. E. Van Horn, 'Changes? What changes? The view of the European patients' movement', *International Journal of Social Psychiatry*, vol. 38, no. 1, pp. 30–5; V. Lindow, Self-help Alternatives to Mental Health Services (London: Mind Publications, 1994).
15. A. Milroy and R. Hennelly, *Changing our Ways* (Chesterfield: Mental Health Services Project, 1985).
16. W. Wolfensberger, 'Social Role Valorisation: a proposed new term for the principle of normalisation', *Mental Retardation*, vol. 21 (1983), pp. 234–9.
17. D. Brandon, 'Implications of Normalisation Work for Professional Skills', in S. Ramon (ed.), *Beyond Community Care: Integration and Normalisation Work* (London: Macmillan, 1991), pp. 35–55.
18. J. Segal, 'The Professional Perspective', in S. Ramon (ed.), *Beyond Community Care: Integration and Normalisation Work* (London: Macmillan, 1991), pp. 85–114.

19. P. Youll and C. McCourt Perring, *Raising Voices* (London: HMSO, 1994).
20. F. Janssen, *Introducing Quality Assurance in a DISH Housing Scheme*, Innovation Project Report, Diploma 'Innovation in Mental Health Work, London School of Economics, August 1994.
21. S. Ramon, 'The Workers' Perspective: living with ambiguity, ambivalence and challenge', in S. Ramon (ed.), *Psychiatric Hospitals Closure: Myths and Realities* (London: Chapman & Hall, 1992), pp. 85–120.
22. J. Segal, 'The Professional Perspective', op. cit., pp. 85–113.
23. L. Swindell, 'Working with Care and Authority: a Groupwork Approach to Child Sexual Abuse', in M. Whitefield (ed.), *Child Sexual Abuse* (London: Family Services Units, 1992).
24. M. Wilson, *Crossing the Boundaries: Black Women Surviving Incest* (London: Virago, 1993); N. Selig, 'Ethnicity and Gender as Uncomfortable Issues', in S. Ramon (ed.), *Psychiatry in Transition* (London: Pluto, 1990), pp. 90–8.
25. S. Ramon, *The Implementation of the NHS and Community Care Act: Views of Frontline Mental Health Social Workers* (Birmingham: British Association of Social Workers, 1993).
26. K. Jones and A. Poletti, 'Understanding the Italian Experience', *British Journal of Psychiatry*, vol. 146 (1985), pp. 341–7.
27. F. Basaglia, 'Breaking the Circuit of Control', in D. Ingleby (ed.), *Critical Psychiatry* (Harmondsworth: Penguin, 1981), pp. 184–92; O. De Leonardis, D. Mauri and F. Rotelli, *L'impresa sociale* (Milan: Anabasi, 1994); M. T. Battaglino, 'Cooperatives de travail et desinstitutionalisation a Turin', in C. Louzoun (ed.), *Sante Mentale: Realites Europeennes* (Paris: Eres, 1993), pp. 243–6.
28. N. Schepher-Huges and A. Lovell (eds), *In and Out of Psychiatry: Selections from Franco Basaglia's Writings* (New York: Columbia University Press, 1987).
29. L. Burti and L. Mosher, *Community Mental Health: Principles and Practice* (New York: Norton, 1989).
30. M. Savio, 'Psychiatric nursing in Italy: an extinguished profession or an emerging professionalism?', *International Journal of Social Psychiatry*, vol. 37, no. 4, pp. 293–9.
31. R. Mezzina, P. Mazzuia, D. Vidoni and M. Impagnatiello, 'Networking consumers' participation in a community mental health service: mutual support groups, citizenship, coping strategies', *International Journal of Social Psychiatry*, vol. 38, no. 1, pp. 68–73.
32. C. Amado, 'Hospitalieser les schizophrenes?', in M. Reynaud (ed.), *Le Traitement des Schizophrenes* (Paris: Frison-Roche, 1991), pp. 203–25; R. Castel, F. Castel and A. Lovell, *The Psychiatric Society* (New York: Columbia University Press, 1982); R. Castel, *The Psychiatric Order* (Cambridge: Polity, 1988); G. Deleuze and F. Guattari, *A Thousand Plateaus: Capitalism and Schizophrenia* (London: Athlone, 1988); F. Guattari, *The Molecular Revolution: Psychiatry and Politics* (Harmondsworth: Penguin, 1984).
33. M. McCrone and G. Strathdee, 'Needs not Diagnosis', *International Journal of Social Psychiatry*, vol. 40, no. 2, editorial.

34. D. Brandon and A. Brandon, *The Yin and Yang of Care Management* (Cambridge: Anglia University, 1993); H. Brown and H. Smith (eds), *Normalisation: A Reader for the 1990s* (London: Routledge, 1992); S. Ramon, (ed.), *Beyond Community Care: Normalisation and Integration Work* (London: Macmillan, 1991).
35. K. Bridges, P. Huxley and J. Oliver, 'Psychiatric Rehabilitation: Redefined for the 1990s', *International Journal of Social Psychiatry*, vol. 40, no. 1 (1994), pp. 1–16.
36. J. Williams, G. Watson, H. Smith, J. Copperman and D. Wood, *Purchasing Effective Mental Health Services for Women: A Framework for Action* (Canterbury: University of Kent, 1993).
37. D. Brandon and N. Towe, *Free to Choose* (London: Good Impressions, 1991).
38. T. Wainwright, 'The Changing Perspective of a Resettlement Team', in S. Ramon (ed.), *Psychiatric Hospitals Closure: Myths and Realities* (London: Chapman & Hall, 1992), pp. 3–47.
39. M. Barnes, R. Bowl and M. Fisher, *Sectioned: Social Services and the 1983 Mental Health Act* (London: Routledge, 1990).
40. M. Sheppard, *Mental Health – the Role of the Approved Social Worker* (Sheffield: Social Services Monographs, University of Sheffield, 1990).
41. S. Ramon, *The Implementation of the NHS and Community Care Act*, op. cit.
42. K. Jones and A. Poletti, 'Understanding the Italian Experience', op. cit., pp. 341–7.
43. F. Basaglia, 'Crisis and Identity', in S. Ramon, (ed.), *Psychiatry in Transition* (London: Pluto, 1990), pp. 252–60; S. Ramon, 'The Reactions of English-Speaking Professionals to the Italian Psychiatric Reform', *International Journal of Social Psychiatry*, vol. 35, no. 1, pp. 120–8; B. Vincente, M. Vielma, A. Jenner, R. Mezzina and J. Lliapas, 'Attitudes of Professional Mental Health Workers to Psychiatry', *International Journal of Social Psychiatry*, vol. 39, no. 2 (1993), pp. 131–41.
44. J. Shears, 'Passive Participants: Social workers' responses to the closure of a psychiatric hospital', unpublished PhD thesis, London School of Economics, 1994.
45. S. Ramon, 'Psichatria Democratica: A case study of an Italian community mental health service', *International Journal of Health Services*, vol. 13 (1983), pp. 307–324; S. Ramon, 'The Workers' Perspective', op. cit., pp. 85–121
46. I. Carino and S. Petri, 'Community Action in Giugliano', *Community Development Journal*, vol. 19 (1984), pp. 89–95; T. J. Peters and R. H. Waterman, *In Search of Excellence: Lessons from America's best-run companies* (New York: Harper & Row, 1984)
47. P. Brown, *The Transfer of Care* (London: Routledge, 1985).
48. K. Darton, J. Gorman and L. Sayce, *Eve Fights Back* (London: Mind Publications, 1994), pp. 23–33.
49. R. Bentall, 'Cognitive Models', in M. Romme and S. Escher (eds), *Accepting Voices* (London: Mind Publications, 1993), pp. 171–6;

238 References

G. Haddock and R. Bentall, 'Focusing', in M. Romme and S. Escher *Accepting Voices*, op. cit., pp. 211–14.
50. S. Holland, 'Psychotherapy, oppression and social action: gender, race and class in black women's depression', in R. Perlberg and A. Miller (eds), *Gender and Power in Families* (London: Routledge, 1992), pp. 256–69.
51. A. Ryle, *Cognitive Analytic Therapy: Autonomy and Control* (Chichester: Wiley, 1991).
52. A. Ryle and H. Beard, 'The integrative effect of reformulation: Cognitive analytic therapy with a patient with borderline personality disorder', *British Journal of Medical Psychology*, vol. 66, no. 3 (1993), pp. 249–74.

7 A Scandalous Category

1. R. Winnick, 'The Image of Mental Illness in the Mass Media', in W. Gove (ed.), *Deviance and Mental Illness* (Beverly Hills: Sage, 1982), pp. 225–46.
2. G. Gerbner, 'The "Mainstreaming" of America: Violence Profile no. 11', *Journal of Communication*, vol. 30, no. 3 (Summer 1980), pp. 10–29.
3. I. F. Brockington, P. Hall, J. Levings and C. Murphy, 'The Community's Tolerance of the Mentally Ill', *British Journal of Psychiatry*, vol. 162 (1993), pp. 93–9; P. Hall, I. F. Brockington, J. Levings and C. Murphy, 'A Comparison of Responses to the Mentally Ill in Two Communities', *British Journal of Psychiatry*, vol. 161 (1993), pp. 99–108.
4. G. Cumberbatch and D. Howitt, *A Measure of Uncertainty: The Effects of the Mass Media* (London: Broadcasting Standards Council, 1989).
5. G. Cumberbatch and R. Negrine, *Images of Disability on Television* (London: Routledge, 1992).
6. S. Moscovici and R. Farr (eds) *Social Representations* (Cambridge: Cambridge University Press, 1984).
7. D. Jodelet, *Madness and Social Representations* (Hemel Hampstead: Wheatsheaf, 1991).
8. D. Adlam, 'TV Crazy', MsC thesis in social psychology, London School of Economics, 1989.
9. S. Cohen, *Folk Devils and Moral Panics* (Oxford: Oxford University Press, 1980), p. 9.
10. H. Hally, 'The mentally ill in the community – folk deval of the nineties?', unpublished MsC dissertation in social policy, London School of Economics, June 1994.
11. J. Fiske, 'Popularity and ideology: A Structuralist Reading of Dr. Who', in W. D. Rowland and B. Watkins (eds), *Interpreting Television: Current Research Perspectives* (Beverly Hills: Sage, 1984), pp. 165–98.

12. J. Hartley, 'Encouraging Signs: television and the power of dirt; speech and scandalous categories', *Australian Journal of Cultural Studies*, vol. 1, no. 2, (1983), pp. 62–82; E. Leach, *Culture and Communication* (Cambridge: Cambridge University Press, 1976).
13. J. Hartley, *Tele-Ology: Studies in Television* (London: Routledge, 1992).
14. Z. Bauman, *Intimations of Modernity* (London: Routledge, 1992).
15. I. Goffman, *Asylums* (New York: Doubleday Anchor, 1961); T. Scheff (ed.), *Labelling Mental Illness* (Englewood Cliffs, NJ: Prentice- Hall, 1975).
16. O. Gillie, 'Matricide points to Schiozphrenia', *The Independent*, 20 August 1987.
17. F. Rotelli, 'Changing Psychiatric Services in Italy', in S. Ramon (ed.), *Psychiatry in Transition* (London: Pluto, 1990), pp. 182–90; O. De Leonardis, D. Mauri and F. Rotelli, *L'impresa Sociale* (Milan: Anabasi, 1994).
18. L. Cancrini and A. Tazza, 'Che cose questa follia?', *Sapere*, February 1984, pp. 10–16; D. Kemali, M. Maj, F. Veltro, P. Crepet and S. Lobrace, 'Sondaggio sulle opinione degli italiani nei riguardi dei malati di mente e della situazione dell'assitenza psichiatrica', *Revista Sprimentale di Freniatria*, 1989 pp. 1301–46.

Name Index

Accepting Voices 60
  Addington, D. and J. 229
    (nn. 49, 50, 51)
Adlam, D. 53, 190
African 75, 79, 82–3
  Afro-Caribbean 75–7,
    78–9, 82–3, 96, 117
Agrigento 204
Ainey-le-Chateau 140–2
Alcoholics Anonymous
  (AA) 34–5
Arezzo 139, 203
Ashworth special hospital
  119, 164
Asian 8, 76–7, 82–3, 88, 96, 117
Asylum Magazine 211
Athens 78
Australia 37, 124
Austria 12, 177

Barnes, M. 41, 223 (n. 21),
  224 (n. 22), 237 (n. 39)
Basaglia, F. (1968) 216 (n.
  21); (1980) 215 (n. 18);
  (1981) 236 (n. 27); (1987)
  100; (1990) 237 (n. 43);
  (1992) 235 (n. 9)
Battaligno, M.T. 234 (n. 43),
  236 (n. 27)
Battersea Project 95
Beard, H. 184
Belgium: foster families 139;
  hospital beds 26;
  legislation 25; mental
  health facilities 3, 28;
  mental illness rate, 10;
  suicide figures, 12
Bentall, R. 219 (n. 27), 238
  (n. 49)
Berlin 96, 156
Birch, A. 150
Birchwood, M. 117
Bosnia 74–5, 178
Brandon, A. 237 (n. 34)
Brandon, D. (1974) 231 (n. 1);
  (1989) 230 (n. 67); (1991
  and N. Towe, *Free to
  Choose*) 237 (n. 37); (1991
  'Implications of
  Normalisation Work for
  Professional Skills) 170,
  222 (n. 60), 235 (n. 17);
  (1991 *Innovation without
  Change?*) 235 (n. 12);
  (1992) 230–1 (n. 67);
  (1993) 237 (n. 34)
Brazil 3
Breakwell, G. 46–7, 218 (n. 8)
Breggin, P. 122
Brel, J. 212
Bridges, K. 237 (n. 35)
Brinck, U. 107, 216 (n. 20),
  217 (n. 25)
Briscoe, M. 90
Britain (UK): assertive
  out-reach programmes

124; challenging behaviour 58; citizen participation 67; community supervision orders 119; comparison with Italy 21; continued care clients 44, 47–8, 104, 107, 108, 118–19; demonisation campaign 49–52, 191; ethnicity 75–9; funding and costs 29, 36, 37, 42; gender issues 91; health service management 167; hearing voices 60; hospital beds 26, 29; hospital policies 28; hospitals 108; legislation 18, 25, 39, 42, 51, 119, 167, 179–80; media coverage 196–200, 208, 209; mental health services 3; mental health task force 19; mental illness rate 10; professional workers 167, 176–7, 179–81; quality assurance 171; registration policy 18, 51; relatives' groups 104, 129; reprovision 35, 37; resettlement 115; role of social workers 41; schizophrenia 56; sexual abuse 64; special hospitals 111–14; suicide figures 10; support services 152; therapeutic communities 146; user movement 67, 134, 165; violence issue 183; welfare services restructuring 22–3; work cooperatives 155
British Medical Association (BMA) 80
British Mental Health Act (1959) 59
British Mental Health Foundation 10
British National Schizophrenia Fellowship 104, 119, 129
British Network for Alternatives to Psychiatry 133
British Royal College of Psychiatrists 96, 117, 119, 121
Brixton Prison 137
Bromsgrove 188
Brown, G.H. 57, 96
Brown, H. 219 (n. 21), 226 (n. 13), 237 (n. 34)
Budapest 34
Buddhism 80, 82
Bulgaria 12
Burti, L. 216 (n. 22), 229 (n. 46), 236 (n. 29)
Busfield, J. 25, 219 (n. 25), 220 (n. 41), 224 (n. 24)

Canada 37, 41, 134
Castel, F. 216 (n. 25), 236 (n. 32)
Castel, R. 236 (n. 32)
Catholic Church 12
CEFEC (Confederation of European Firms, Employment Initiatives and Co-operatives for the Psychically Disabled) 159
Central League for Mental Health (Finland) 131

Name Index

Chamberlayne, P. 215 (n. 17), 225 (n. 35)
Chamberlin, J. 216 (n. 21), 231 (n. 72)
Chesterfield Support Network *see* Tontine Road Mental Health Project
Chinese 79
Ciompi, L. (1981) 218 (n. 4); (1982) 55; (1985) 108; (1994) 57, 219 (n. 29), 220 (n. 35)
Ciponi, E. 58
Client Union 131
Cohen, S. 50, 190–1
Colegno 1
Confucianism 81
Conlan, E. 217 (n. 27)
Copenhagen 96
'Coping with Violence and Aggression: Prevention and Management' 118
Costanzo, M. 206
Council of Europe 6, 9, 10, 21
Crepet, P. (and Lofrenzano, 1988) 224 (n. 22); (Kemali, Maj, Veltro, Lobrace and, 1989) 239 (n. 18); (1990) 216 (n. 20), 218 (n. 15); (and Ferrari, Platt and Bellini, 1990) 10; (1994) 225 (n. 39)
Croatia 95, 178
Cumberbatch, G. 188, 238 (nn. 4, 5)
Cyprus 78
Czechoslovakia 3, 12, 108

Daily Express 190–1
Daily Mail 49
Davies, L.M. 37
Davis, A. 87
de Jonge, M. 151, 233 (n. 34)
De Leonardis, O. 234 (nn. 41, 42), 236 (n. 27), 239 (n. 17)
De Plato, G. 100, 226 (nn. 8, 9), 231 (n. 71), 232 (n. 15)
Denmark 3, 10, 12, 39, 52, 124
Diekstra, R.F.W. 10, 213 (n. 7, 9), 214 (n. 13, 17)
Drummond, M.F. 37
Dublin 156
Dur-sur-Arun 140
Durkheim, E. 13
Dutch User Movement 151

England 12, 26, 39
English National Board 118
Escher, S. 60–2
European Mental Health Regional network 6
European Regional Council 132
European Union (EU): CEFEC 159; employment initiatives 154; financial contribution 154, 157; impact 6; membership 2; mental health policies 20–1; mental illness statistics 10; Slovenia initiative 177; *see also* Council of Europe
European Users Network 21, 103–4, 132, 227 (n. 18), 231 (n. 75)

FAF (Forderung in Arbeitinitiativen und Firmenprojekten) 158
Fanon, F. 81–2

Fanon Project 83
Farkas, M.D. 120
Fellini, F. 205
Finland: hospital beds 26; mental health facilities 3; mental illness rate, 10; suicide rates, 11, 12; users' groups, 104
Finnish Mental Health Association 130–1
Foucault, M. 53, 179
France: assertive out-reach programmes 124; continued care clients 44, 47, 124; ethnicity 75, 79; health service funding 23; hospital beds 26; legislation 25; mental health facilities 3; mental health policies 28, 30; prison prevention structure 111; professional workers 167; psychosis 100; reformers 175; social psychiatric projects 45; suicide figures 12; work cooperatives 155
Francis, E. 81, 223 (nn. 14, 16)
Fernando, S. 213 (n. 3), 219 (n. 25), 222 (nn. 3, 4)
Fountain Club 152
Freedom to Care 163–4, 235 (n. 5)
Freud, S. 63–4, 184
Furlong, R. 99, 218 (n. 13)

Garmezy, N. 70
Gerbner, G. 188
Germany: assertive out-reach programmes 124; continued care clients 44, 47, 124; employment projects 156, 158; ethnicity 79; funding and costs 23, 30, 37, 42, 171; hospital beds 26; legislation 25; mental health facilities 3; professional workers 167; schizophrenia 56; social psychiatric projects 45; suicide rate, 11, 12; user groups 165; work cooperatives 156
Gheel, Belgium 139, 142
Gilligan, C. 222 (n. 3)
Glennerster, H. 235 (n. 10)
Goffman, I. (1961) 46, 194, 239 (n. 15), 216 (n. 21), 218 (n. 10); (1963) 219 (n. 25)
Goodwin, S. 25
Grassroots 19
Greece: community mental health centres 26; hospital beds 26; hospitals 108, 109, 140; legislation 39; long-term users 106; mental health facilities 3; mental health service restructuring 21; migrants and mental illness 78; nurses 101; schizophrenia 56; suicide figures 12
Grove, T. 107
Grulisaco 1
Guardian 196, 199
Gypsies 35

Hally, H. 191, 228 (n. 41)
Hamid, W. 231 (n. 1)

Name Index

Hantrais, L. 215 (n. 9)
Harmat, P. 11
Harris, T. 57, 96
Harrison, G. 77
Hartley, J. 239 (nn. 12, 13)
Hatfield, A. 221 (n. 52), 227 (n. 16), 231 (n. 68)
Health of the Nation 107
Hearing Voices Networks 61
Helsinki 131
Hennelly, R. 169
Henry, P. 218 (n. 3)
Hiday, V. 228 (n. 42)
Higgins, Dr 199
Hill, R. 27, 216 (n. 20), 234 (n. 36)
Hinduism 80
Hirsch, S. 56
Holland, S. 81, 223 (nn. 16, 17), 225 (n. 45), 238 (n. 50)
Holloway, F. 217 (n. 1), 221 (n. 53), 227 (n. 19), 229 (n. 53), 230 (n. 60)
House of Commons Select Health Committee 51
Howitt, D. 188
Hungary 3, 11–13, 33–5, 108
Hungerford massacre 196–200, 207
Huntly Lodge, Glasgow 147
Husband, C. 222 (nn. 1, 3)
Huxley, P. 237 (n. 35)

Iceland 12
Imola 175
Independent 18, 117, 196, 199
Institute of Psychiatry, London 37
Ireland 10, 12, 39, 140, 156
Irish 75–6, 79
Islam 81

Italian Mental Treatment Law (1978) 25, 200
Italy: assertive out-reach programmes 124; care coordination 125; continued care clients 44, 47, 101, 104, 108, 115, 124–5; funding and costs 36, 42; gender issues 85; guardianship 41; health care cooperatives 31; health service funding 23; hospital beds 26, 29; hospital closures 26, 27, 28, 32, 50, 191; legislation 25; media coverage of reform 200–1; media coverage of mental distress 201–6, 208–9; mental health facilities 3; mental health rate 10; normalisation 52; nurses 101; professional workers 161, 163, 167, 180; reformers 1, 100, 172–5, 177, 181; rehabilitation schemes 21, 115; relatives' groups 104, 129; schizophrenia 56, 196; social role valorisation 52–3; special hospitals 111, 114; suicide figures 12; user groups 104, 132, 165; violence 117–18; work cooperatives 156

Jack, R. 13, 88–9, 214 (nn. 15, 20, 22)
Jahoda, M. 8
Japan 3
Jewish 79, 84

Name Index 245

Jewish Care 84
Jodelet, D. 140–2, 190, 213 (n. 4)
Johnson, T. 234 (n. 2)
Jones, D. 221 (n. 54), 226 (n. 1), 227 (n. 17), 235 (n. 9)
Jones, K. 180, 215 (n. 16), 236 (n. 26)
Jones, M. 100, 215 (n. 16)

Kashenko hospital, Moscow 31–3
Kent University 37
Kiev 1, 128–9, 154–5
Klein, M. 102
Knapp, M. (and Beecham, 1992) 233 (n. 19); (and Cambridge, Thomason, Beecham, Allen and Darton, 1992) 37–8, 217 (nn. 29, 31), 228 (n. 37), 232 (n. 18), 235 (n. 11)
Krietman, N. 10, 213 (n. 6, 10), 214 (n. 14, 16)

Lahti 131
Lambo Centre, The 83
Law 180 *see* Italian Mental Treatment Law (1978)
Lawrence, M. 224 (n. 30), 225 (n. 42), 229 (n. 43)
Lawson, M. 219 (n. 24)
Leff, J. 5, 56, 220 (nn. 30, 31, 34)
Leros 21, 109, 140
Levander, M. 100
Limburg University 60–1
Lindow, V. (1991) 224 (n. 32); (1993) 211, 231 (n. 79); (1994) 67, 221 (n. 50), 134, 231 (n. 78), 224 (n. 32), 235 (n. 14)
Lisbon 164

Littlewood, J. 221 (n. 58)
Littlewood, R. 223 (nn. 10, 11, 17)
Ljublijana 178
London 20, 82, 96, 149, 155, 161, 172, 178, 195
London Women's Therapy Centre 95
Louzoun, C. ('New and Old Mental Health European Realities' 1993) 5; (*Sante Mentale* 1993) 25, 213 (n. 1), 226 (n. 6), 227 (n. 28), 229 (n. 46), 236 (n. 27)
Luxembourg 12, 39

McCannell, E. 110, 114
McCourt Perring, C. (1992) 45, 168, 227 (n. 24), 228 (n. 37), 232 (n. 17); (Youll and, 1994) 236 (n. 19)
McCreadie, R.G. 110, 114
McCrone, M. 5, 237 (n. 33)
Machin, S. 164
Madianos, M.G. 21
Mafia 204
Malta 12
Malvern 188
Manchester 156
Mangen, S. 25, 213 (n. 1), 215 (nn. 14, 15), 216 (nn. 19, 20, 25), 222 (n. 6)
Mason, B. 95
Mason, E. 95
Masson, J. 63, 230 (n. 55)
Mattinson, J. 149
Maurizio Costanzo Show 203–7
Mental Health Act (1959) 39
Mental Health Act Commission 39–40, 217 (n. 34), 228 (n. 32)

Mental Health Foundation
213 (n. 5), 216 (n. 23)
Mental Health Specific Grant
scheme 36
Methodist Church 32
Mezzina, R. 227 (n. 27), 228
(n. 35), 232 (nn. 8, 16), 236
(n. 31), 237 (n. 43)
Milan 50
Milroy, A. 169
Mind 115
Minuchin, S. 95
Morgan, S. 229 (n. 46), 235
(n. 8)
Moscow, Kashenko hospital
31–3
Mosher, L. 215 (n. 18), 216
(n. 22), 229 (n. 46), 236
(n. 29)
Muijen, M. 229 (n. 53), 230
(n. 59
Mullender, A. 221 (n. 58),
225 (n. 44)
Murphy, E. 228 (n. 41), 233
(n. 30)

Nafsiyat 78, 83
NAMI 128–9, 155
Naples 50, 94, 96
National Foundation of
Patients and Residents
Council 131
National Mental Health Task
Force 19, 48
Nehring, J. 234 (n. 36)
Neighbourhood Project 95
Netherlands: advocacy
projects 29, 45, 131;
assertive out-reach
programmes 124; care
coordination 125; care
programming 42;
continued care clients 44,
47, 104, 108, 111; ethnicity
78; health service funding
23, 29, 31, 48; hearing
voices 60; hospital beds
26; hospitals 71, 108, 111;
mental health facilities 3;
pressure groups 48;
quality assurance 171;
relatives' organisations
129; suicide rate 12;
support schemes 152;
user organisations 67,
104, 165
New Zealand 134
NHS and Community Care
Act (1990) 22, 177
Norway 10, 12
Nottingham 145
NSF *see* British National
Schizophrenia Fellowship
Nuova Cooperativa, La 156

O'Brien, M. 90
O'Donoll, M. 37
Oliver, J. 237 (n. 35)
Onyett, S. 229 (n. 45), 230
(n. 62)

Parma 156
Pecs 34
Pembroke, L.R. 221 (n. 51),
224 (nn. 30, 32)
Perlberg, R. 223 (n. 16), 225
(nn. 36, 46), 230 (n. 56),
238 (n. 50)
Petch, A. 232 (n. 18), 233 (n. 23)
Pilgrim, D. 222 (n. 4), 228
(n. 36), 233 (n. 26)
Piro, S. 100

Platt, S. (1984) 224 (n. 22), 225 (n. 41); (1986) 221 (n. 53); (and Krietman, 1990) 10, 213 (nn. 6,10), 214 (nn. 14, 16); (Crepet, Ferrari, Bellini and, 1992) 213 (n. 8); (Diekstra, Maris, Schmidtke, Sonneck and, 1989) 213 (n. 7)
Poland 12, 132
Poletti, A. 180, 236 (n. 26)
Pordenone 156–7
Portugal 3, 10, 12, 31, 101, 108, 164
Powell, Enoch 19
Prato self-help group 132, 175, 231 (n. 76)
Protestant Church 12
Psycho-Social Services, Germany (PSS) 149
Purchasing Effective Mental Health Services for Women: A Framework for Action 94

Ramon, S. (1983) 237 (n. 45); (1985) 214 (n. 5), 220 (n. 41), 224 (n. 28); (*Psychiatry in Transition*, 1990) 25, 218 (n. 3), 224 (n. 24), 225 (n. 45), 226 (n. 7), 228 (n. 35), 236 (n. 24), 237 (n. 43), 239 (n. 17); ('Relevance of Symbolic Interaction Perspectives...' 1990) 218 (n. 9); (1991) 218 (n. 11), 219 (nn. 21, 24), 221 (n. 60), 230 (n. 58), 233–4 (n. 35), 235 (nn. 17, 18), 237 (n. 34); (*Care Management*, 1992) 230–1 (n. 67); (*Psychiatric Hospitals Closure*, 1992) 214 (n. 4), 216 (n. 22), 217 (n. 28), 218 (n. 6), 227 (n. 24), 232 (n. 17), 235 (n. 13), 236 (n. 21), 237 (n. 38); (1993) 227 (n. 15), 236 (n. 25), 237 (n. 41); (1995) 234 (n. 42)
Recomincare di Essere 1
Reconstructing Schizophrenia 55
Residential Care Allowance 147
Richmond Fellowship 146
Rogers, A. 222 (nn. 4, 7), 223 (n. 10), 228 (n. 36), 233 (n. 26)
Romania 19
Rome 50, 156, 203, 205–6
Romme, M. 60–3, 238 (n. 49)
Roosnes, E. 139
Rose, N. 53, 219 (nn. 23, 25), 220 (n. 41), 224 (n. 28)
Rotelli, F. 100, 234 (n. 41), 236 (n. 27), 239 (n. 17)
Royal College of Physicians 119
Russia 3, 31–3, 108
Ryan, M. 197–8, 207, 208
Ryle, A. 184, 230 (n. 56), 238 (nn. 51, 52)

Sanctuary, The 83
SANE (Schizophrenia, A National Emergency) 50, 119, 195, 218 (n. 17)
Saraceno, B. 100
Sasso, C. 205
Savio, M. 201, 226 (n. 10), 234 (nn. 42, 44, 3), 236 (n. 30)
Scheff, T. 194, 219 (n. 25)

Name Index

Scotland 12, 39, 110
Scott, J. 137, 232 (nn. 2, 5)
Scott, R.D. 229 (n. 45)
Scull, A. 216 (n. 24)
Segal, J. (1991) 170, 172, 218 (n. 11), 221 (n. 60)
Shanti 83, 96
Shashidran, S. 81, 223 (nn. 14, 16)
Shepherd, G. 150
Sheppard, M. 87, 237 (n. 40)
Sinason, V. 102, 219 (n. 26), 221 (nn. 46, 47), 230 (nn. 56, 57)
Singer, M. 56
Siris, S.G. 121–2, 229 (n. 51)
Slovenia: ethnicity and gender issues 74–5, 86, 95; hospitals 26, 86, 106; mental health facilities 3, 108, 169, 177–9; nurses 101
Social Chapter 20
Social Fund 154
Social Rehabilitation Association 100
Soglia, L. 129
SOS Service 131
Southall Black Sisters 83, 96
Spain 3, 10, 12, 30, 39, 56
Special Scar, A 69
Spicker, P. 214 (n. 2)
SSO (Survivors Speak Out) 133, 211
Strathdee, G. 5, 229 (n. 43), 237 (n. 33)
Strutti, C. 215 (n. 11), 216 (n. 20), 227 (n. 25)
'Survivor, Activist or Witch' 134
Svab-Cotic, V. 216 (n. 20), 224 (n. 23), 227 (n. 21)
Swain, J. 218 (n. 7)

Sweden: community mental health centres 26; continued care clients 100, 104, 107; gender issues 85; hospital beds 26; legislation 39; mental health policies 26, 30; mental illness rate 10; normalisation 52; suicide figures 12; users' organisations 104, 132
Switzerland 12, 44, 45, 156

Tavistock Institute of Marital Relations 149
Telegraph, The 196, 197, 199
Tempus 178
'Ten Thousand Sheets Later' 205
Thatcher, M. 198
Thomas, C. 77, 222 (n. 5)
Thornicroft, G. 226 (n. 1), 229 (n. 43), 233 (n. 19)
Times, The 194, 196, 198, 199
Tomlinson, D. 217 (n. 28), 235 (n. 9)
Tonight 191
Tontine Road Mental Health Project 91
Trieste 97, 143, 145, 156–7, 161, 175
Trieste University 139
Trieste Women's Space 95
Turin 1, 50, 96, 146, 156, 202
Turkish 79
Tuscany 175, 203

Ukraine 1, 3, 108, 155
Unicef 19
United Kingdom (UK) *see* Britain

United States: assertive out-reach programmes 124; care coordination 125; community mental health centres 30; community supervision orders 41, 119; continued care clients 30, 44, 98; cost studies 37; demonisation campaign 49–51; drug therapy study 39; ethnicity 78; hospital policies 28; housing schemes 138; media 201; mental health facilities 3; mental health policies 1–2, 7, 28, 30–1, 183; mental health task force 19, 20; normalisation principle 52; public administration 176; relatives' groups 104; schizophrenia studies 196; support services 152; user movement 67, 131, 134
van de Graaf, W. 71
van der Meer, D. 71
van Hoorn, E. 134, 231 (nn. 74, 80), 235 (n. 14)
van Weeghel, J. 153, 229 (n. 47), 230 (nn. 63, 66), 233 (n. 34), 234 (n. 38)
Voices 104

Wainwright, T. 216 (n. 22), 217 (n. 28), 237 (n. 38)
Wales 12, 26, 39
Wallace, M. 50, 52, 194–6
Warner, R. 99, 230 (n. 58), 233 (n. 35)

Water Towers 19
Wertheim, A. 69
White City Women in Mental Health Project 83, 95
Williams, D. 49
Williams, J. 94, 237 (n. 36)
Wilson, M. 236 (n. 24)
Wing, J.K. (1972) 230 (n. 64); (1978) 213 (n. 1); (1981) 218 (n. 4); (1982) 218 (n. 14), 232 (n. 6); (and Furlong, 1986) 99, 218 (n. 13); (Thornicroft, Berwin and, 1992) 233 (n. 19); (Wykes and, 1991) 228 (n. 38)
Winnick, R. 188, 238 (n. 1)
WISH (Women In Special Hospitals) 113, 228 (n. 34)
Wolf, J. 229 (n. 47), 230 (nn. 63, 66)
Wolfensberger, W. 176; (1972) 219 (n. 19); (1979) 221 (n. 57), 222 (n. 3); (1983) 52–3, 219 (n. 20), 235 (n. 16); (Kugel and, 1969) 218–19 (n. 19)
World Health Organisation (WHO) 6, 10, 12, 14, 19
World Mental Health Federation (WMHF) 21
Wykes, R. 218 (n. 14)
Wykes, T. 228 (n. 38), 231 (n. 1), 232 (n. 6)
Wynne, L.Y. 56

Ytantopolous, J. 21, 227 (n. 20)
Yugoslavia 12, 20, 75

Zeelen, J. 71, 153, 233 (n. 34)

Subject Index

abuse: child 91, 95; ethnicity 172; gender issues 88, 91, 95, 96; sexual 44, 63–6, 88, 91, 95, 96, 102, 123, 147, 172, 184; survivors' support groups 96; women users 89; work with survivors 102, 123, 172, 184
action research 70–1, 182
advocacy: British schemes 36, 131; European schemes 120; need for 4; Netherlands schemes 29, 45, 131; pressure groups 48; Slovenian position 178; support groups 96
affect logic 55, 57
age 12, 16, 211
AIDS 92
alcohol abuse 14, 34–5, 86
alternative interventions 82–4
anorexia *see* self-harm
approved social workers (ASWs) *see* social workers
assertive out-reach 30, 123–4
assessment 5, 20, 165–6, 177, 180

brokerage 128, 176

care: coordination 125–8; management 23, 36, 42, 48, 120, 125–8, 166–7, 169, 177; programming 23, 42
CAT *see* psychotherapy
challenging behaviour 58–60; accommodation 139, 144; British units 35; deconstruction 44; gender issue 91; hospital placements 139; professional responses 184
change, radical 18
communication, family style 56
community care 24, 37, 42, 52–3; costs 38 (Table 1.2)
community mental health centres: European policy 17, 106, 120; gender issues 96; Greek provision 21, 26; Italian 139; legislation 25; special hospital dischargees 114; Swedish provision 26; US programme 30
community supervision orders 41, 51, 59, 119
compulsory admissions 76, 86, 87, 129, 180; legislation 39–41
continued care clients (long-term users) 44–52, 98–135; community care

250

Subject Index

effectiveness studies 37; Italian reform 174; professional intervention 162; rediscovery of 5, 174, 104–6; US programme 30; user movement 67, 130–5
cost: accommodation 144; British community care 37–8 (Table 1.2); cutting 17, 30, 35; drug therapy 37, 39; effectiveness 17, 35, 37; measurement 36–7; registration 18; unemployment effects 149
counselling 122–3, 125, 168, 180

day care, day activities: British 115, 148; continued care clients 115, 116, 148; ethnic support services 84; European provision 106, 120; Italian 115; Slovenian 178; US programme 30; work opportunities 150
dehospitalisation 5, 25–9, 30–1, 35–6, 44, 46–7
deinstitutionalisation 29–36, 44, 130
demarginalisation 44, 45
demonisation 6, 45, 49–51, *see also* folk devils
depression: gender issues 86, 91, 93, 96; intervention strategies 56, 184–5; medication 99, 121–2; schizophrenia 55; special hospitals 113; suicides 13–14, 119; support services 152

deviancy school approach 190–1
disability: accommodation 146; carers 90; drug therapy 37, 39; French reforms 175; legislation 42; marginalisation 16; movement 45–6; Social Chapter programme 21; social role valorisation 52–3; value judgements 98, 189
Down's Syndrome 157
drug therapy *see* medication

efficiency 17
elderly 16; *see also* age
electroconvulsive therapy (ECT) 40
employment: discharged inpatients 114–15; gender issues 89; needs 4, 148–54; projects and schemes 116, 120, 154–8, 159, 165, 169, 178; *see also* unemployment
ethics 70
ethnicity 73–84; British task force 19; central identity marker 73–7; continued care clients 116–17; intervention methods 6; mental health ethics 4; minorities 45; 'new long stay' 49; racism 74, 76–7, 81, 209; schizophrenia 76–7, 117; sexual abuse 172; statistical information 9; support structures 93, 96; 'threatened identity' 46

Subject Index

expressed emotions 44, 55–7, 124

family: communication style 56; placements 139–42; *see also* relatives
folk devils 50, 191; *see also* demonisation

gender: carers and clients 24, 89–90; central identity marker 73–5; conceptual innovations 92–3; continued care clients 116; depression 57; in Europe 84–5; interventions 6, 93–7; men and mental distress 90–2; mental distress and 85–9; mental health service ethics 4; 'new long stay' 49; statistical information 9; suicide incidence 13; survivors' groups 211; women users 89; women's movement 45
gentle teaching 53
group homes 142–5, 168
groupwork, self-directed 94–5
guardianship 40–1, 180

hearing voices 60–3, 67, 71
HIV 92
homelessness: court diversion scheme studies 112; increased 22; in Italy 111; mental illness 6, 50, 136–8, 158; 'new long stay' 116, 209

hormonal treatment 40
hospitals: bed numbers 26 (Table 1.1); closure processes 17, 599; closures in England 19, 27 (Figure 1.1); closures in Italy 44, 52, 181; closures in Europe 5; continued care clients 98, 99–100, 106, 107–11; deinstitutionalisation 29–36; discharge from 114–16, 144; ethnicity 75; funding 6, 36–9, 48; gender issues 89, 96; Greek programme 21; hostels 138–9; inpatients 107–11; leaving 46; legislation post-1980 39; legislation pre-1980 25; media coverage of Italian scandal 204; policies post-1980 25–9; policies pre-1980 24–5; private 6; professional workers 160–1; psychiatrists 99–100; readmission 144; registration policy 18; rehabilitation programmes 104; relatives' initiatives 129; special 111–14; suicide issues 11; therapeutic communities 146; violence 183; *see also* dehospitalisation
housing: community care costs 38 (Table 1.2); community living 30; core and cluster schemes 145–7; employment and

149; ethics 4; ethnic support services 84; gender issues 89; group homes 142–5; hospital hostels 138–9; individualised tenancies 147–8; mental illness 23; needs and wishes 136–8; schemes 131, 138, 145–7; sheltered 106, 115, 165; solutions 138–42, 158–9; supported 120; therapeutic communities 146–7; *see also* homelessness

immigrants 77–8, 88, 96
income 4, 30, 120
innovation: British scheme 36; concept of 70–1; gender issues 92–3, 95; professional responses 169, 178–80, 185
insurance, health 23, 29, 31, 171
Italian psychiatric reform 172–5; approach to mental illness 100; celebration of achievements 1; desegregation of hospitals 152; effects 208–9; involvement of health workers 181; media coverage 200 1; media coverage of mental distress 201–3; rediscovery of continued care clients 48; resettlement in community 52; violence 117–18

labelling 59, 63, 88
learning difficulties: challenging behaviour 58–9; French 'family colony' 190; psychoanalytic approach 102, 123, 184; relatives' organisations 129; sexual abuse 64, 65; social role valorisation 54
legislation: British 18, 25, 39, 42, 51, 119, 167; gender issues 84; liberal 5; post-1980 39–42; pre-1980 25; reflection of policy 16; social security issues 159
legitimation crisis 18–19
long-term users *see* continued care clients

marginalisation 16
media: analysed examples 190–1, 194–206; conceptual framework 187–94; 'dirt' 192, 196–7, 199, 203, 204, 207; methodological implications 189–194; role 17–18, 43, 186–7, 207–9; sensationalism 49–50, 51, 183; 'scandalous category' 192, 202, 206, 208
medication 120–2; alternatives 6, 63, 68, 212; assertive out-reach 124; Clozapine 37, 39; costs and benefits 37, 39; employment issues 151, 155; ethnicity 75; gender

medication (*cont.*)
    issues 89, 94, 96; hearing voices 60; hospital regime 109; legislation 119; 'new long stay' 49; not taking 49, 51, 111, 116, 118; overuse 67–8, 80, 89; psychotropic drugs 98–9, 103; questioning usefulness 6; schizophrenia 99; suicide 11
men *see* services for men
mental distress and illness 8–10; gender issues 85–93; hearing voices 61–2; Hungarian approach 33; integrative approach 69–70; media approaches 193–4; medication 99; migration 77–8; national rates 10 (Table 1); non-Western approaches 81; normalisation 52–3; Portuguese approach 31; relatives' groups 125; social role valorisation 52–4; statistics 106; understanding of 31, 47
mental health task force 19, 48

new long stay: characteristics 49, 98, 115–16; demonisation 51, 209; housing needs 145, 147; inpatients 107–8; Italian policy 111; resettlement 25
normalisation 45, 52–3, 102, 150, 176, 179

nurses: gender issues 87; in Italy 175; legal issues 40; power relations 71; roles 148, 160, 182, 183; training 67, 118, 182; view of long-term users 101

occupational therapy 24, 34
old long stay 98, 107, 209
out-reach *see* assertive out-reach

participation 94
police 76
positivist content analysis 187–9
poverty 22, 23
power relationships 71, 166–70, 179–83
prisons 111–12, 137, 209
professional roles 160–85
professionalism 71
psychiatric classification: affect logic 57; biological approach 8; challenging behaviour 58–60; clients and workers 105–6; deconstruction 44, 54–7; gender issues 87; hearing voices 60–3; role of diagnosis 5, 47, 184
psychiatrists: challenging behaviour concept 59; critique of hospitals 28; deconstruction process 54–5; Eastern European 33–5; ethnic issues 79–81; gender issues 87, 96, 161; legal issues 25, 40, 119; mental health policies 24; neighbourhood role 182,

183; office 171; power relations 71, 161, 180; prison diagnoses 112; psychosocial approaches 5, 96; role in Italy 48, 94, 174–5; schizophrenia approaches 76, 119, 121–2; Slovenian 169, 178; suicide policy 14; view of long-term users 99–101
psychoanalysis *see* psychotherapy
psychoeducation 124–5
psychologists: challenging behaviour concept 59; deconstruction process 54; Eastern European 33, 34; gender issues 87; neighbourhood role 182; psychosocial approaches 5; reform approaches 184; sexual abuse issues 63–4; special hospitals 113; suicide policy 14; view of long-term users 102
psychopathy 59
psychosurgery 40
psychotherapy: alternative interventions 82–4; CAT 184–5; clients and workers 105–6; cognitive behavioural approaches 54, 184; continued care clients 122–3; counselling 122–3, 125, 168, 180; family therapy 54, 95, 125, 130, 175, 184; gender issues 95; Greek community 78; Hungarian approaches 34–5; learning difficulties 184; psychoanalysis 54, 63–4, 95, 100, 102, 123, 170, 175, 184; reforming 184; relatives' organisations 129–30; role 165; self-harm 11, 120
purchasers and providers 94, 177

quality assurance 138, 171

race *see* ethnicity
racism 74, 76–7, 81, 209
rediscovery of continued care clients 47–8
reformers 175–9, 184; *see also* Italian psychiatric reform
refugees 74–5, 96, 178
rehabilitation: assertive out-reach 123–4; British programme 44, 176; continued care clients 104; employment 153; ethnic minorities 75; Greek provision 106; housing 150; inpatients 110; 'new long stay' 116; policy focus on 27–8, 100, 120, 129; relatives' influence 48, 129; Slovenian programme 178; US programme 30, 44; user groups 130
relatives 68–9; carers 24, 89; consultation 167–8; continued care clients 14, 103, 104; influence 43, 44, 66; Italian media presentation 202; murder cases 118; 'new long

relatives (*cont.*)
stay' 116; organisations 104, 128–30, 155; own initiatives 128–30; rehabilitation 48; schizophrenia 70; self-harm 11, 119; working with 124–5
reprovision 35–7
resettlement: accommodation 115, 158; British approach 176–7, 209; challenging behaviour 59; continued care clients 104; in Italy 52, 173; non-family settings 25; 'old long stay' 49, 115; outcome statistics 50; professional workers' views 181; reprovision 36
resilience factors 70
risk 53, 68, 117, 180, 183

salutogenic factors 70
schizophrenia: affect logic 57; approaches 55–7; concept 5, 55; deconstruction 44; demonisation campaign 49–50; diagnostic label 5, 58; ethnicity 76–7, 117; family relationships 70; gender issue 86; hearing voices 60; media presentation 194–6, 199–200, 207; medication 99, 119, 121–2; 'new long stay' 49; numbers 107; relatives' initiatives 128–9; self-harm 13–14, 116; Swiss study 45; women on remand 112
self-directed groupwork 94–5
self-harm 51, 60, 68, 74, 88, 113, 116, 119–20, 132, 152, 184; anorexia 68, 88, 91, 96, 116, 119; attempted suicide 10–11, 13–14, 88, 92, 119, 145; suicide 10–15 (Table 2), 69, 91, 92, 110, 116, 119, 145, 162, 212
services for men 91, 93–4, 96, *see also* gender
services for women 5, 84, 93–7, 113, 129; *see also* gender
sexual abuse *see* abuse
sexuality 74, 89
social policies 16–43, 44: formation processes 16–20; context 20–4; mental illness 18–19, 42; pre-1980 24–5; post-1980 25–9; poverty programme 20; welfare debate 22–3, 42, 176; *see also* deinstitutionalisation, dehospitalisation
social representation 189–90
social role valorisation (SRV) 52–4; assertive out-reach programmes 124; British reformers 176; emergence of concept 44; ethics 70; housing 129, 150; impact 67; in Italy 52–3, 129; psychologists' views 102; social workers' training 180; work cooperatives 155

Subject Index 257

social workers and approved social workers (ASWs): deconstruction process 54; ethnicity issues 76; gender issues 87; hospital critique 28; legal issues 40–1, 161; media portrayal 195; professional roles 179–82; psychosocial approaches 5; Slovenian 178–9; suicide policy 14; user movement training 67; view of long-term users 102–3
special hospitals 80, 89, 111–14, 119, 164
stakeholders 2–4, 8, 19, 28, 35, 44, 66, 70, 98; politicians 43; carers 19; professionals (professional identity, roles, power issues) 43, 71, 99–103, 160–85; professionals (responses to change) 171–2, 174, 180–2, 184–5; relatives 66–8; workers 19; users 19, 43, 44, 66–8, 71, 103–4, 107–11
statistics 9–12; demonisation campaign, 50; gender issues, 85; Mind survey 115; outpatients 106–7 (Table 4.1); schizophrenia and ethnicity 117; Scottish inpatients, 110, 114; special hospitals, 111
suicide *see* self-harm

therapeutic communities 146–7
threatened identity 46, 67, 69, 94

unemployment 13, 22–3, 77, 91–2, 149–50, 153; *see also* employment
users' organisations 130–5

violence to others: demonisation campaign 49–51; gender issues 91; handling 132, 183, 212; media coverage 196–200, 207–8; 'new long stay' 116; risk of 117–19, 162; special hospitals 114; user movement approach 68; *see also* self-harm
voices, hearing 60–3, 67, 71

welfare policies 22–4
whistle blowing 163–4, 204
women *see* gender, services for women